PSYCHIATRY SPECIALTY BOARD REVIEW

BRUNNER/MAZEL CONTINUING EDUCATION IN PSYCHIATRY SERIES

Series Editor: Gene Usdin, M.D.

This series provides comprehensive, state-of-the-art study guides to help those who are preparing for advanced examinations in psychiatry. Written by experts representing various areas of specialization, the guides are designed to be accurate, current, and accessible.

Brunner/Mazel Continuing Education in Psychiatry Series No. 1

PSYCHIATRY SPECIALTY BOARD REVIEW

William M. Easson, M.D.

Professor of Psychiatry
Division of Infant, Child, and Adolescent Psychiatry
Louisiana State University Medical Center
New Orleans, Louisiana

Nicholas L. Rock, M.D.

Professor of Clinical Psychiatry
Division of Infant, Child, and Adolescent Psychiatry
Louisiana State University Medical Center
New Orleans, Louisiana

Medical Director
The Rock Creek Foundation
Silver Spring, Maryland

BRUNNER/MAZEL PUBLISHERS • NEW YORK

Notice: As our knowledge in clinical sciences is constantly changing, new information becomes available, and changes in treatment and in the use of drugs become necessary. The authors and the publisher of this volume have taken care to make certain that the doses of drugs and schedules of treatment are correct and compatible with the standards generally accepted at the time of publication. However, the reader is advised to be fully cognizant of the instruction and information material provided in the package insert of each drug or therapeutic agent before administration. This admonition is essential, especially when using new or infrequently used drugs.

Library of Congress Cataloging-in-Publication Data
Easson, William M.
    Psychiatry specialty board review / William M. Easson, Nicholas M. Rock.
        p.   cm. — (Brunner/Mazel continuing education in psychiatry series ; no. 1)
    Includes bibliographical references.
    ISBN 0-87630-617-2
    1. Psychiatry—Examinations, questions, etc.   I. Rock, Nicholas L.   II. Title.   III. Series.
    [DNLM: 1. Psychiatry—examination questions.   WM 18 E13pc]
RC457.E183   1991
616.89 ′0076—dc20
DNLM/DLC
for Library of Congress   90-15116
                                                                 CIP

Published by
BRUNNER/MAZEL, INC.
19 Union Square West
New York, New York 10003

Manufactured in the United States of America

10 9 8 7 6 5 4 3 2 1

CONTENTS

FOREWORD

This is a stimulating, constructive work that provides a most important service for psychiatrists and neurologists preparing for their specialty Boards, the PRITE, the FLEX, or other examinations. Easson and Rock have built upon their experience in helping to develop questions for Part I of the American Board of Psychiatry and Neurology examinations as well as upon their participation over many years as examiners for the Oral Board examinations.

This volume provides a "dry run" experience to help familiarize psychiatrists and neurologists with the format and type of questions used in the Part I examination. This "rehearsal" is a major asset of the review, as the response style necessary for successful examination performance should improve with practice and familiarity. Although many of the questions in this book are likely to appear in the Board examinations, this volume is not meant to be a "crib sheet," anticipating only the questions that will be asked.

Apart from those preparing for Board examinations, psychiatrists and neurologists in general will find this book challenging and worthwhile. It provides an update on the state of our knowledge, and for many, it will serve as a reminder of the need for additional reading or a refresher course. References are provided with each answer, thus facilitating further study.

Psychiatry is experiencing an explosion of new knowledge and information. Staying current has become a formidable task. Many clinicians feel overwhelmed—to paraphrase Toffler—by the acceleration of the rate of new knowledge production. The half-life of new information in psychiatry and medicine continues to become increasingly brief, so that the physician who relies simply on the medical knowledge acquired during residency soon finds this knowledge base out-of-date.

The advanced degree of knowledge required to answer the questions in this volume is impressive; even well-read psychiatrists and neurologists will be challenged by the contents. Clinicians who carefully work through this text will become well informed about current psychiatry.

—GENE USDIN, M.D.
Senior Psychiatrist, Ochsner Clinic
Clinical Professor of Psychiatry
Louisiana State University Medical School
New Orleans, Louisiana

PREFACE

When we were students, we may have looked forward to that day when examinations would be finished. Increasingly, however, political and professional pressures have made Board certification almost obligatory; now Board certification is to be time limited and recertification will be required. Examinations will be with us throughout our professional lives.

This book is designed to prepare the clinician for the written examinations for Board certification and recertification and for the Psychiatry Resident in Training Examination. Psychiatrists, physicians in other specialties, and nonphysicians can use this book to update psychiatric knowledge. The types of questions on the topics that are likely to appear in the PRITE and Board examinations are presented in the format used in these examinations. To facilitate more extensive review, all questions are referenced to the current editions of three standard psychiatric textbooks.

One of us (W.E.) prepared the questions, the other (N.R.) wrote the answers, and together we reviewed all of the components of the book. We came to appreciate that some questions used in these examinations are vague, controversial, and lacking clear scientific validity and some require answers that are of dubious validity and based on limited or uncertain data. The textbook references are at times equally vague and confusing, and frequently reflect opinion rather than fact; occasionally the textbooks disagree on the answers provided. Periodically, our own clinical experience has not supported the answers given. In the questions and answers, we have tried to indicate areas where there is uncertainty and disagreement.

In the formal examinations, the questions are not presented in any specific topic area, but in this book we have grouped subject areas together for easier review and more efficient learning. Where the answer to a question is fairly specific, we have not repeated in the answer the data given in the question, but have provided supplementary information.

As we have limited the questions in this book to those that are referenced in the most recent textbooks, we do not cover journal publications in the last two years. For a complete examination update, the reader should also review the general psychiatric journals that have appeared in the last two or three years to ascertain what is current and fashionable, and the subjects of recent discussion that are likely to be examination topics.

In preparing this book, we have learned a great deal. Above all, we have come to appreciate the wide range of topics that the examination candidate is expected to know. To each and every reader, we wish examination success and a deeper understanding of both the knowledge base of our specialty and of questions yet to be formulated and answered.

WILLIAM M. EASSON
NICHOLAS L. ROCK

REFERENCES

Throughout this book, each question and chapter is referenced to three psychiatry textbooks. Rather than list each textbook and its authors with each reference, we have cited them as CTP, APA, and Har at the end of each answer.

CTP: Harold I. Kaplan and Benjamin J. Sadock, *Comprehensive Textbook of Psychiatry/V*, Fifth Edition, Williams & Wilkins, Baltimore, Md., 1989.

APA: John A. Talbott, Robert E. Hales, and Stuart C. Yudofsky (Ed), *Textbook of Psychiatry*, The American Psychiatric Press, Inc., Washington, D.C., 1988.

Har: Armand M. Nicholi (Ed), *The New Harvard Guide to Psychiatry*, Belknap Press of Harvard University Press, Cambridge, Mass., 1988.

PDR: *Physicians' Desk Reference*, 44th Edition, Medical Economics Company, Inc., Oradell, N.J., 1990.

PSYCHIATRY SPECIALTY BOARD REVIEW

1

CHILD AND ADOLESCENT PSYCHIATRY

DIRECTIONS: Select the single best response for each of the questions 1–50.

1. According to Piaget, a major achievement of the sensorimotor period is:

    1. Object constancy
    2. Object permanence
    3. Object relations
    4. Object symbolization
    5. Object conservation

2. A mother complains that her 20-month-old child is demanding and unpredictable. One moment he is clinging to her, asking to be held or carried; the next moment he is darting away out of her sight. According to Mahler's developmental theory, the child is now showing behavior characteristic of the phase of:

    1. Symbiosis
    2. Differentiation
    3. Practicing
    4. Rapprochement
    5. Object constancy

3. Stranger anxiety:

    1. Occurs when the child is separated from the mother
    2. Is present at about 2 months of age
    3. Indicates that the child can differentiate between caregiver and others
    4. Is more marked when the child has had multiple caretakers
    5. Indicates developmental pathology

4. The earliest sign of puberty in a normally developing girl is usually:

    1. Development of axillary hair
    2. Onset of menses
    3. Breast bud development
    4. Appearance of pubic hair
    5. Rapidly increasing height

5. The onset of puberty in a normally developing male is usually first indicated by:

    1. Increase in testicular volume
    2. Increase in size of hands and feet
    3. Upper lip hair
    4. Increase in muscle mass
    5. Enlargement of the larynx

6. All of the following are normal developmental events except:

    1. Transitional object
    2. Stranger anxiety
    3. Separation anxiety
    4. School phobia
    5. Symbiosis

7. The latency period is characterized by:

    1. Prominent fear of castration
    2. Parental rules internalized in the superego
    3. Resurgence of incestuous feelings
    4. Preoccupation with sadistic themes
    5. Frequent imaginary companions

8. According to Kohut's theory of development, mirroring is:

    1. Interaction whereby the child defines him- or herself by observing the mother's response
    2. A process whereby the infant mimics the mother's behavior
    3. The infant's preambivalent splitting into good and bad mother images
    4. A pathological process leading to "as if" personality
    5. An outward manifestation of infantile hallucinatory omnipotence

9. When you take your car in for repair, the mechanic lists the possible causes of your problem and the methods that will be used to find the defect. According to Piaget, this thinking is an example of:

    1. Concrete operations
    2. Circular reactions
    3. Preoperational representation
    4. Formal operations
    5. Sensorimotor intelligence

10. You take your car to a mechanic for repair. He states that it may be problem A and tests this out, but your car still does not work. He suggests then that it may be problem B, makes an adjustment to deal with this, but with no success. After several tries, he hits on the problem, corrects it, and you drive your car away. The me-

chanic's thinking is an example, according to Piaget, of:

1. Sensorimotor intelligence
2. Preoperational representation
3. Concrete operations
4. Formal operations
5. Circular reactions

11. You give a child a collection of blocks of different sizes and ask him to arrange them in order of size. He piles up the small blocks together and the larger blocks in another heap, but seems unable to arrange them in a row, gradually increasing in size. His arrangement of the blocks indicates:

    1. Formal operations
    2. Probable mental retardation
    3. Appreciation of conservation
    4. Preoperational thinking
    5. Understanding of seriation

12. A mother asks your advice as to how she should best manage her 2-year-old son. For several months he has been carrying around an increasingly soiled teddy bear. He screams and cries if anyone tries to take this tattered toy from him. You advise:

    1. Take away the toy and destroy it
    2. This is normal behavior, and he will give up the toy eventually
    3. This is an early manifestation of autistic withdrawal
    4. The child is showing signs of emotional deprivation
    5. This is a reaction to castration anxiety

13. Gender identity is established by:

    1. Age 1 year
    2. Age 3 years
    3. Age 6 years
    4. Age 9 years
    5. Onset of puberty

14. Infant temperament:

    1. Predicts long-range behavioral patterns
    2. Is unchangeable
    3. Is important in the way it fits with parents
    4. Is easily measured
    5. Shows clear sex differentiation

15. Character traits related to the anal stage include all of the following except:

    1. Neatness
    2. Punctuality
    3. Ambivalence
    4. Dependency
    5. Stubbornness

16. Erikson used the concept "integrity" to refer to:

    1. The controlling, restraining force of conscience
    2. The ability to maintain loyalties
    3. The wisdom and stability of old age
    4. The ability to promote growth
    5. The trust of a mutually caring relationship

17. The anal phase, according to classical Freudian theory, corresponds to the Erikson stage:

    1. Industry versus inferiority
    2. Initiative versus guilt
    3. Intimacy versus isolation
    4. Autonomy versus shame
    5. Integrity versus despair

18. A 2-year-old child is left alone for a few minutes while the mother goes upstairs. On mother's return, an emotionally secure child is liable to:

    1. Hit at mother, telling her she was "naughty"
    2. Hold her skirt briefly and then return to play
    3. Ignore her, continuing to play
    4. Stop playing and insist on being held for the next half hour
    5. Have a tantrum

19. According to Bowlby, a young child reacts to mother's departure with:

    1. Protest, despair, detachment
    2. Denial, anger, bargaining, depression
    3. Denial, intellectualization, reinvestment
    4. Shock, anger, displacement
    5. Clinging, crying, rage

20. All of the following statements are true about mentally retarded children except:

    1. Most are not recognized at birth as being retarded
    2. Most do not become progressively less competent
    3. Most do not have unusual head size
    4. Most require institutional placement eventually
    5. Most are mildly retarded

21. All of the following statements about lead encephalopathy are correct except:

    1. Commonly presents with visual hallucinations
    2. Most frequent in young children
    3. Associated with pica
    4. Subjects are often irritable and clumsy
    5. Treated with calcium disodium edetate

22. True statements about elective mutism include all of the following except:

    1. Commonly starts in preschool
    2. Associated with profound deafness
    3. Persistently refuses to speak in specific social situations

4. Often stubborn and resistant

5. May communicate with gestures

23. All of the following statements about burn patients are true except:

1. High incidence of alcohol and drug abuse

2. Psychiatric prognosis is better for children compared with adults

3. Frequently delirium due to electrolyte imbalance

4. Depression, anxiety, and phobic behavior are common in first year after burn

5. Most patients, previously healthy emotionally, recover fully psychiatrically

24. In treating a 9-year-old enuretic child with imipramine, all of the following are correct except:

1. Bedtime dose of 25 mg is usually adequate

2. Will take 2–4 weeks to have effect

3. Often causes sleep disturbance and nightmares

4. Relapse rate is high after discontinuation

5. Improvement is not due to anticholinergic effect

25. All of the following statements about children with attention deficit hyperactivity disorder are true except:

1. Higher incidence in Tourette's disorder

2. Patients grow out of symptoms at puberty

3. Most often diagnosed in grade school

4. Show different levels of hyperactivity in different settings

5. Usually have normal intelligence

26. The five stages of adaptation to dying described by Kubler-Ross:

1. Occur in clearly predictable sequence

2. Those patients who work through all stages benefit emotionally

3. Are not specific to dying, but occur with other losses

4. Include fear, anxiety, and denial

5. Are present from age 5

27. All of the following apply to fetal alcohol syndrome except:

1. Mental retardation

2. Low birth weight

3. Small head size

4. Infantile cirrhosis

5. High infant mortality

28. Severe mental retardation is:

1. Commonly due to sociocultural deprivation

2. One to two percent of retarded population

3. More often due to autosomal than sex chromosome abnormality

4. Not commonly associated with emotional disorder

5. Frequently caused by Down's syndrome

29. When methylphenidate is used in the treatment of children with attention deficit hyperactivity disorder, side effects include all of the following except:

1. Insomnia

2. Abdominal pain

3. Headaches

4. Enuresis

5. Loss of appetite

30. Male, mildly retarded, long narrow face, enlarged testes indicate:

1. Down's syndrome

2. Phenylketonuria

3. Hurler's disease

4. Fragile X syndrome

5. Galactosemia

31. Reactive attachment disorder:

1. Occurs after a child, age 6–12 months, is separated from a competent caregiver

2. Reflects markedly inadequate caregiving

3. As described by Bowlby, is a response to prolonged separation from the infant's mothering person

4. Is an early manifestation of infantile autism

5. Is a severe form of stranger anxiety

32. In cases of child abuse, the following statements are correct except:

1. Most child abusers are women

2. The abusing parent is likely to say that the abused child is different

3. The abusing parent is often psychotic

4. The abusing parent rationalizes the abuse as being necessary discipline

5. Most abused children are under age 3

33. The following statements about sexual abuse of children are valid except:

1. There is increased incidence of multiple personality disorder in these children

2. Victim may develop post-traumatic stress disorder

3. In most cases the child was involved in a single abuse episode

4. Most abusers are known personally by the victim

5. The victim is frequently depressed and suicidal

34. In an evaluation session with a friendly 6-year-old boy, the child begins a game with playhouse dolls in which a boy doll keeps pushing two adult dolls out of the bedroom. The most helpful way to deal with this play would be to:

1. Ask him why he is angry with the father doll
2. Describe the dolls' emotions without interpreting
3. Wonder how the boy doll felt about the bedroom activities
4. Suggest that the angry boy doll felt castrated or threatened
5. Encourage the behavior of the boy doll

35. Factors predicting continuation of childhood antisocial behavior into adult life include all of the following except:

    1. Onset before age 10
    2. Involvement with delinquent peers
    3. Greater number of antisocial behaviors
    4. Greater range of situations where antisocial behavior is manifested
    5. Childhood psychiatric hospitalization

36. Nightmares in childhood:

    1. Usually persist into adult life
    2. Occur during stage 3–4 sleep
    3. Are associated with panic disorder
    4. Are more frequent towards the end of night
    5. Result in the youngster's being confused and agitated

37. One to two hours after falling asleep, a 5-year-old boy wakens, crying, screaming, and stating that "a bad man was coming to get me." With reassurance, he goes back to sleep. This recurs several times in the next three months. This behavior is likely to be:

    1. Sleep terror disorder
    2. Overanxious disorder
    3. Panic disorder
    4. Dream anxiety disorder
    5. Adjustment disorder with anxious mood

38. Nightmares and night terrors:

    1. Both indicate psychopathology
    2. Both occur in non-REM stage 3–4 sleep
    3. Both are more common in males
    4. Both have morning amnesia
    5. Both have maximum incidence in grade-school years

39. The following statements about night terrors in childhood are correct except:

    1. They are more common in males
    2. They are most frequent in grade-school children
    3. Morning amnesia is usual
    4. They occur during REM sleep
    5. There is usually no causative psychopathology

40. When compared with girls, in grade school ages 7–12, boys are likely to be:

    1. Academically superior
    2. Better coordinated physically
    3. Taller
    4. Showing other-sex characteristics
    5. Less interested in other-sex friends

41. Your neighbor is very upset and ashamed because her 3-year-old son took off his pants at school. You advise her that this behavior is:

    1. An indication that he has been sexually molested, possibly at school
    2. A manifestation of infantile masturbatory drives
    3. An age-appropriate reaction to castration anxiety
    4. Age-appropriate undersocialized behavior
    5. Evidence of gender role confusion

42. When a colleague refers a 16-year-old patient with anorexia nervosa, you anticipate that all of the following will be true except:

    1. The patient is female
    2. The patient has amenorrhea
    3. The patient has a normal dexamethasone suppression test
    4. The patient enjoys preparing food
    5. The patient abuses laxatives

43. In patients with anorexia nervosa, all of the following are true except:

    1. Higher incidence in people who jog
    2. Better prognosis with late onset
    3. Higher incidence in family members
    4. Purging may lead to cardiac arrhythmias
    5. Frequently decreased sexual interest

44. All of the following syndromes are more commonly diagnosed in boys than in girls except:

    1. Elective mutism
    2. Stuttering
    3. Attention deficit hyperactivity disorder
    4. Mild mental retardation
    5. Tourette's disorder

45. A 20-year-old patient with identity disorder is likely to show all of the following except:

    1. Depression and sleep disturbance
    2. Uncertainty over a career choice
    3. Conflict about gender identity
    4. Doubts about religious affiliation
    5. Conflict about selection of friends

46. In deciding which parent in a divorce suit should have the custody of a child, the decision is usually based on:

    1. The financial resources of each parent
    2. The child's stated preference

3. The emotional stability of each parent
4. The best interest of the child
5. The social and academic resources that exist where the parent lives

47. The following statements about children with autistic disorder are correct except:

    1. The majority of these patients test at the retarded level
    2. Hallucinations are common in preadolescence
    3. Patients are most commonly male
    4. Seizures often develop by adolescence
    5. There is increased incidence in siblings

48. All of the following statements about developmental reading disorder in children are correct except:

    1. More common in males
    2. Results in generally lower IQ
    3. Often associated with conduct disorders
    4. The children usually have spelling problems
    5. Disability likely to persist into adulthood

49. Conduct disorder in childhood is associated with all of the following except:

    1. Antisocial personality in adulthood
    2. Attention deficit hyperactivity disorder
    3. Poorer prognosis with early onset
    4. Lower incidence of suicidal behavior
    5. Property crime arrests peak at age 16

50. The mind-altering drug most often used by American high school seniors is:

    1. Marijuana
    2. Cocaine
    3. Alcohol
    4. Cigarettes
    5. Amphetamines

DIRECTIONS: For questions 51 through 130, one or more of the alternatives given are correct. After you decide which choices are correct, record your answer according to the following.

(A) if alternatives 1, 2 and 3 only are correct.
(B) if alternatives 1 and 3 only are correct.
(C) if alternatives 2 and 4 only are correct.
(D) if alternative 4 only is correct.
(E) if all four alternatives are correct.

51. According to Kohlberg's schema of moral development, which of the following apply to the post-conventional stage of morality?

    1. It is attained during the latency period
    2. Moral cues are external, motivation is internal

3. Motives are to avoid punishment
4. Rules of society are relative rather than absolute

52. According to Spitz's genetic field theory, organizers in the development of child behavior include:

    1. Smiling response
    2. Stranger response
    3. "No" response
    4. Shame response

53. According to Spitz, the "No" response:

    1. Indicates separation emotionally from mother
    2. Reflects beginning of conscience development
    3. Occurs during the toddler phase
    4. Signifies the beginning of concrete operational thinking

54. Separation anxiety:

    1. Develops about age 4 months
    2. Indicates that the child can distinguish mother from others
    3. Is a precursor of conscience development
    4. Is more intense when the attachment to the caretaker is more intense

55. According to Ainsworth, the fear of an 18-month-old child in a stranger situation can be reduced if:

    1. The stranger approaches directly and quickly
    2. The stranger picks up the child and cuddles
    3. The parent leaves the child with the stranger
    4. The parent is present

56. Stranger anxiety:

    1. Normally occurs at age 12–15 months
    2. Occurs when the child differentiates caregivers from others
    3. Predicts separation anxiety disorder
    4. Represents fear and curiosity of strangers

57. By 2 months of age, a normal infant:

    1. Becomes fearful of strangers
    2. Coos and gurgles in response to social stimulation
    3. Becomes anxious when separated from the mother
    4. Follows objects across the midline

58. By age 1 year, a normally developing child:

    1. Points to what he wants
    2. Builds a tower of four blocks
    3. Imitates adult speech sounds
    4. Walks downstairs with hand held

59. A 3-year-old child should be able to:

    1. Copy a square
    2. Give her full name
    3. Name three colors correctly
    4. Take turns

60. According to Mahler, object constancy:

    1. Occurs at age 12–15 months
    2. Leads to primitive conscience development
    3. Marks resolution of stranger anxiety
    4. Relieves separation anxiety

61. During the rapprochement phase of development (Mahler):

    1. The youngster can leave and return to the mother
    2. The toddler needs the reassurance of mother's presence
    3. The child recognizes his separation from mother
    4. The child first shows stranger anxiety

62. In testing a child, you start with two same-size containers, each containing the same amount of liquid. You pour one into a short, wide flask and the other into a tall, narrow flask. When the child is asked to choose, she picks the tall, narrow container, because, she says, "it contains more." When the youngster is asked how previously equal amounts can become different, she says, "I don't know." Her thinking according to Piaget:

    1. Is in the preoperational stage
    2. Shows concrete operational stage
    3. Is typical of a 5- or 6-year-old
    4. Recognizes conservation of mass

63. A normally developing 2-year-old child is able to:

    1. Alternate feet going down stairs
    2. Use three-word sentences
    3. Wait to take turns
    4. Build a seven-block tower

64. A normal 18-month toddler can:

    1. Imitate mother sweeping
    2. Pull up pants
    3. Carry out two requests
    4. Copy a circle

65. In Winnicott's developmental theory, the following are important normal developments:

    1. Good enough mothering
    2. Infantile omnipotence
    3. Transitional objects
    4. Basic trust

66. Toilet training is best carried out after a child is 18 months of age because:

    1. Early coercive training leads to enuresis or encopresis
    2. Gastrocolic reflex begins to operate
    3. Punishment is not effective with young children
    4. Child wants to please parents

67. Gender identity is:

    1. Secondarily resolved during early adolescence
    2. Decided by external genitalia
    3. Settled by the resolution of the oedipal conflict
    4. Determined primarily by social learning

68. Characteristics of early childhood temperament identified by Chess and Thomas include:

    1. Rhythmicity
    2. Threshold of responsivity
    3. Activity level
    4. Speed of adaptation

69. Categories of infant temperament described by Chess and Thomas include:

    1. Dysrhythmic
    2. Quick to respond
    3. Short attention
    4. Slow to warm up

70. Attitudes and character traits related to the anal stage of development include:

    1. Orderliness
    2. Frugality
    3. Stubbornness
    4. Curiosity

71. During the oral phase, the following occur:

    1. Development of ambivalence
    2. Establishment of object constancy
    3. Establishment of primitive superego
    4. Development of object relationships

72. According to S. Freud, the Oedipus complex in boys:

    1. Leads to the castration complex
    2. Reawakens at puberty
    3. Has a major influence on psychosexual orientation
    4. Finally stabilizes object constancy

73. The Oedipus complex in girls, in classical Freudian theory:

    1. Follows and is initiated by the castration complex
    2. Leads to the castration complex
    3. In its resolution has major influence on the superego
    4. Occurs only in early neurosis

74. Inadequate caregiving during infancy increases the risk for:

1. Childhood behavior disorders
2. Physical growth retardation
3. Academic failure
4. Infantile autism

75. The stage of intimacy versus isolation according to Erikson:

   1. Coincides with the Freudian latency period
   2. Deals with the issue of heterosexual bonding
   3. Focuses on problems of retirement
   4. Occurs during young adulthood

76. In a normally developing child, which of the following are expected motor skill landmarks?

   1. 2-year-old can copy a cross
   2. 3-year-old can copy a circle
   3. 4-year-old can copy a diamond
   4. 5-year-old can copy a square

77. A 3-year-old child should have the following skills:

   1. Can take turns
   2. Copies a circle
   3. Knows up, down, front, back
   4. Knows two colors correctly

78. In evaluating a child's suicidality, it is important to know:

   1. History of suicidal behavior in the family
   2. The child's concept of death
   3. The parental reaction to the child's behavior
   4. The child's mood

79. In dealing with adolescent suicide, which of the following statements are correct?

   1. Most suicide attempts in adolescence are associated with major depression
   2. Suicide is the most common cause of death in adolescence
   3. The suicide rate is highest in the teenage years and then gradually decreases
   4. Teenage suicide is often associated with conduct disorders and drug abuse

80. The following statements are valid about a child's concept of death:

   1. A 4-year-old child sees death as reversible journey
   2. A 6-year-old child appreciates that death is irreversible
   3. A 7-year-old child tends to see death personified—as a ghost
   4. A 7-year-old child recognizes that death is universal

81. Down's syndrome is associated with:

   1. Trisomy 21
   2. Alzheimer's disease

3. Congenital heart defects
4. Hydrocephalus

82. Which of the following statements apply to Down's syndrome?

   1. There is a high incidence of childhood hearing problems
   2. Most are moderately to severely retarded
   3. There is increased risk of hypothyroidism
   4. It is difficult to find adopting parents

83. Children with moderate mental retardation:

   1. Can reach about the fifth grade academic level by adulthood
   2. Can be trained to take care of themselves
   3. Often are not diagnosed until adolescence
   4. Are able to work in sheltered workshop

84. Which of the following statements about mentally retarded children are correct?

   1. There is increased risk for emotional disorder
   2. They are more often referred for psychiatric treatment
   3. The highest diagnosed incidence is in adolescence
   4. They do not benefit from psychotherapy

85. Increased incidence of mental retardation occurs with:

   1. Maternal alcohol abuse
   2. Maternal retardation
   3. Maternal hydantoin use
   4. Maternal schizophrenia

86. Early diagnosis and prompt treatment reduce or prevent mental retardation in which of the following syndromes?

   1. Cretinism
   2. Lead intoxication
   3. Phenylketonuria
   4. Wilson's disease

87. Pica:

   1. May cause intestinal obstruction
   2. Can lead to toxic encephalopathy
   3. May produce nutritional deficiencies
   4. Has a higher incidence in retarded

88. Which of the following statements about blind children are correct?

   1. They tend to be dependent and insecure, resembling phobic children
   2. After 2 months of age, smile becomes bland due to lack of visual reinforcement
   3. Infants and toddlers are less able to tolerate separation from the mother
   4. Motor development tends to be lower

89. In managing a grade-school child with diabetes mellitus, parents should understand:

    1. Chronic physical illness does not increase the risk of emotional disorder
    2. If possible, the child should be cared for at home rather than in hospital
    3. Anger about the illness worsens the prognosis
    4. A child adapts better when treated realistically by parents

90. Stuttering in grade school children:

    1. Is much more common in boys
    2. Tends to improve spontaneously
    3. Most often begins in preschool period
    4. Has a higher family incidence

91. Functional enuresis:

    1. Has an incidence by age 10 of 0.5–1.0% of boys
    2. Has a higher family incidence
    3. Is more common with harsh training
    4. Is more common in males

92. In teenagers hospitalized with major depression, the best predictors of future bipolar disorder are:

    1. Gradual onset of depressive symptoms
    2. Family history of affective disorder in succeeding generations
    3. Coexistent learning disability
    4. Tricyclic induced hypomania

93. Which of the following statements are correct about conduct disorder and depression in teenagers?

    1. Teenagers with no history of conduct disorder may develop conduct disorder when depressed
    2. Long-standing conduct disorder may lead to major depression
    3. Teenage suicide attempters often have a history of drug abuse and conduct disorder
    4. Serious depression is uncommon with adolescent conduct disorder

94. In dealing with depression in a 13-year-old child:

    1. Earliest manifestation is likely to be depressive themes in child's fantasy
    2. Earliest manifestation would be an abnormal Dexamethasone Suppression Test
    3. Confirmation is best obtained by interviewing child
    4. Confirmation is best obtained by interviewing parent

95. In a normal 4-year-old child, the death of a parent is viewed as:

    1. Punishment for being bad
    2. Reversible and parent will return
    3. Boogyman took parent away
    4. Abandonment

96. Fetal alcohol syndrome results in:

    1. Long narrow face
    2. Delayed growth
    3. Renal hypoplasia
    4. Mental retardation

97. Phenylketonuria:

    1. Autosomal dominant
    2. Blonde hair, blue eyes
    3. Treatment by excluding milk from the diet
    4. Musty smell

98. In considering management of children with attention deficit hyperactivity disorder, it must be recognized that:

    1. Children treated with methylphenidate do much better academically
    2. Children treated with tricyclic antidepressants quickly develop tolerance
    3. Stimulant medication is ineffective in adults
    4. Adult drug abusers have a higher incidence of childhood attention deficit hyperactivity disorder

99. Children with attention deficit hyperactivity disorder:

    1. Tend to be disliked by peers
    2. Have symptoms usually first noted in preschool years
    3. Have a higher incidence in siblings
    4. Have a high incidence of adult personality disorders

100. Which of the following statements about children with attention deficit hyperactivity disorder are valid?

    1. They often have academic problems
    2. They may not show obvious hyperactivity during mental status testing
    3. They frequently have family history of antisocial behavior
    4. There is a higher incidence of somatization disorder in female relatives

101. In the treatment of children with attention deficit hyperactivity disorder, stimulant medication:

    1. Improves academic performance, leading to better grades
    2. Produces rise in achievement on intelligence testing
    3. Leads to long-term improvement in conduct disorder
    4. Reduces inattention and impulsivity

102. When children with attention deficit hyperactivity disorder are treated with methylphenidate, it should be recognized that:

1. Treatment effects are specific to children with this disorder
2. Symptom improvement will persist several weeks after stopping treatment
3. Treatment has beneficial effects on patients with dyslexia
4. Treatment improves social behavior of most children with attention deficit hyperactivity disorder

103. Imipramine used in childhood disorders:

1. FDA-recommended dose not to exceed 5 mg per kilogram weight
2. Lowers seizure threshold
3. May cause aggressiveness and temper outbursts
4. Enuretics frequently become tolerant to medication with the return of symptoms

104. Which of the following are characteristics of abused children?

1. They are more likely to have medical illness
2. They are often aggressive towards their peers
3. They are frequently provocative towards adults
4. They are more likely to have academic difficulties

105. Which of the following statements about child sexual abuse are correct?

1. If the child can give details of alleged sexual molestation and identify the perpetrator, abuse has usually occurred
2. The abuser is usually a person known to the child
3. Child protection agencies must be notified in every case of suspected child abuse
4. In mother-son incest, the mother is usually emotionally ill

106. When psychotherapy with children is compared with psychotherapy with adults, correct statements include:

1. Nonverbal communication is more frequent and more important
2. The child therapist has to be less involved in the therapy
3. The child's capacity for self-observation is more limited
4. Transference reactions are greater for children than adults

107. In the psychodynamic psychotherapy of the preadolescent child, which of the following statements are correct?

1. Violent toys should be excluded from the playroom
2. To maintain trust and confidentiality, parents should be rarely involved
3. The child must be able to verbalize freely
4. Termination often occurs when presenting problems have resolved

108. When children are treated with imipramine, which of the following statements are correct?

1. With attention deficit hyperactivity disorder, beneficial results tend to be immediate
2. Enuretic boys are likely to show relapse when treatment is discontinued
3. With major depression, patients do not develop tolerance
4. Children are less sensitive to cardiotoxic effects

109. When haloperidol is used in the treatment of autistic children, which of the following statements are valid?

1. Lowers appetite, reduces weight gain
2. Reduces stereotypic behavior
3. Liable to induce motor tics
4. Combined with behavior therapy, improves language ability

110. Which of the following statements are correct regarding the use of antipsychotics with children?

1. Tardive dyskinesia does not occur with low-dose, short-term treatment
2. Dystonic reactions usually appear within 72 hours
3. Young children are less likely to develop akathisia
4. Withdrawal dyskinesias may occur when antipsychotic medication is withdrawn abruptly

111. Oppositional defiant disorder:

1. Is most likely to evolve into adult passive aggressive personality disorder
2. Is often specific to certain situations
3. May show behavior normal for a 2- or 3-year-old child
4. Violates the personal rights of others

112. In the management of severe obsessive compulsive disorder in a 13-year-old girl, which of the following treatments could be beneficial?

1. In vivo exposure and response prevention
2. Fluoxetine
3. Family therapy
4. Clomipramine

113. Imaginary companions:

1. Often occur in children age 3–6 years
2. Are more frequent in phobic children
3. Are more likely in socially isolated adults
4. Are a manifestation of separation anxiety

114. Studies of the contact between the mother and the newborn infant show:

1. Higher incidence of child abuse where no contact in the delivery room
2. More disinterested maternal behavior where delayed postnatal contact

3. Delivery room contact had consistent positive effect on mother-child interaction
4. Interest in bonding has caused hospitals to change obstetrics care

115. Psychiatric evaluation should be recommended for a 3-year-old with which of the following symptoms?

1. Imaginary companions
2. Night terrors
3. Nocturnal enuresis
4. Head-banging when angry

116. Thumb-sucking in children:

1. May cause later dental problems
2. Indicates maternal deprivation
3. Is present in most infants
4. Is associated with future teenage depression

117. Separation anxiety disorder in grade-school children:

1. Typically manifests first before age 4
2. Is more common in abused, neglected children
3. With early occurrence has poorer prognosis
4. Occurs in Tourette's disorder treated with haloperidol

118. School absenteeism is often a manifestation of:

1. Conduct disorder
2. Separation anxiety
3. Childhood depression
4. Sociocultural attitudes

119. Manifestations of separation anxiety in grade-school children include:

1. Stomachaches, nausea, tiredness
2. Symptoms primarily from Sunday evening through Friday morning
3. Parents who had similar symptoms
4. Emotionally distant parents

120. Treatment of separation anxiety school absenteeism may include:

1. Tricyclic antidepressant
2. Counseling for parents
3. Early return to school
4. Evaluation of the school environment

121. Which of the following statements apply to patients with Tourette's disorder?

1. Higher incidence in males
2. Higher incidence in relatives of Tourette females than in relatives of males
3. Higher incidence of attention deficit hyperactivity disorder
4. Higher incidence of mental retardation

122. In patients with Tourette's disorder:

1. Symptoms may wax and wane over months
2. Symptoms may be voluntarily suppressed
3. Symptoms are likely to be lifelong
4. Symptoms may be helped by clonidine

123. Effective treatments for Tourette's disorder include:

1. Pimozide
2. Haloperidol
3. Clonidine
4. Carbamazepine

124. Grade-school children with overanxious disorder:

1. Have physical symptoms similar to anxious adults
2. Are best treated with methylphenidate
3. Tend to have anxious parents
4. Are more commonly females

125. In teenagers, borderline personality disorder may be manifested by:

1. Functional encopresis
2. Impulsive rage outbursts
3. Suicidal behavior
4. Substance abuse

126. Increased incidence of autistic disorder is associated with:

1. Congenital rubella
2. Fragile X syndrome
3. Phenylketonuria
4. Infantile spasms

127. Characteristics of children with infantile autism include:

1. Obsessive need for sameness
2. Stereotyped rituals
3. Preoccupation with moving objects
4. Poor eye contact

128. Valid statements about children with infantile autism include:

1. The prognosis is best indicated by the development of social speech
2. The autism is caused by neglectful or rejecting parents
3. Low-dose haloperidol often helpful
4. Its incidence related to socioeconomic class

129. Which of the following statements about anaclitic depression are correct?

1. It is now included in reactive attachment disorder of infancy
2. It is likely to develop during the first three months of life

3. It can be prevented by good nurturing and medical care
4. It occurs after separation when infant has made a normal attachment to mother

130. Normal hallucinations in childhood include:

1. Hypnagogic phenomena
2. Imaginary playmates
3. Eidetic images
4. Lilliputian hallucinations

ANSWERS AND EXPLANATIONS

1. **(2)** *Object permanence* (developed during ages 9–12 months) is, in the sensory-motor Piagetian main period or major stage of cognitive development, the first of four major stages. (*APA 97–98, 101, 131, 1269. CTP 258.*)

   Object constancy is based on Margaret Mahler's separation-individuation theory where, after separation, the child (24–30 months) keeps a stable mental image of the important caretaker.

   Object relations (according to Anna Freud's multilinear theory) is a child's mental representation of significant adults such as parents. *Object integration* refers to affective stability and a synthesis between previously separated good and bad experiences.

   Symbolization is a general mechanism in all human thinking by which mental representation comes to stand for some other thing, a class of things or an attribute.

2. **(4)** *Rapprochement* was described in M. Mahler's subphase 3 of development and represents the child's needs and mixed feelings for closeness alternating with needs for distance. It occurs after child is able to walk and is beginning representational cognition (ages 16–24 months). (*APA 93, 104, 146, 1269. Har 609.*)

   Symbiosis during infancy peaks at 4 to 5 months and is the omnipotent fusion with the representation of the mother, with the delusion of a common boundary for two physically separate individuals. Outside of the normal phase of infant development, symbiosis refers to a mutually reinforcing relationship between two persons who are dependent on each other.

   Differentiation occurs when the infant, around 7–8 months, begins to move away from mother.

3. **(3)** *Stranger reaction*, also called *stranger anxiety*, occurs during the process of the differentiation phase. It is the central theme in this developmental stage and shows how cognitive behavior is associated with cognitive integration; that is, the child realizes the difference between mother and others. (*APA 109, 146.*)

4. **(4)** The first sign of puberty is the development of breast buds and breast enlargement, with increase in size and pigmentation of areolae and nipples at about ages 10–12 years. Growth of pubic and axillary hair occurs later. Height spurt starts at age 11, peaks at 12, then falls off at 14–15 years, two years earlier than in boys. (*APA 113–14, Har 640–41.*)

5. **(1)** Puberty in boys starts with a rise in hormonal output, which first produces increased testicular volume.

Thereafter, pubic hair and axillary hair develop, along with deepening of voice. Increased growth rate of masculine habitus starts at age 12, peaks at 14, and falls off at ages 16–17 years. (*APA 114. Har 641.*)

6. **(4)** In addition to explanations in questions 2 and 3, *transitional objects* were described by D. Winnicott as the infant's first object possession that is perceived as separate from the infant's self and has soothing qualities reminiscent of mother. School phobia, school avoidance, and refusal may be symptoms of separation anxiety disorder or conduct disorder. (*APA 97, 110, 146, 673. Har 188, 608.*)

7. **(2)** During the latency period of development, children normally become concerned and moralistic about rules. (*APA 106. CTP 377–78.*)

8. **(1)** Kohut described *mirroring* as part of development of the cohesive self and included idealization mirroring; the child defines himself by observing himself in the gleam of his mother's eye. (*APA 142. CTP 366–67.*)

9. **(4)** Piaget's fourth major stage is called *formal operations*. He defined four major stages or main periods of cognitive development based on direct child observations in a nonclinical setting. (See question 11 for more details.) First, *sensorimotor* (0–2 years), close connection between body activity and mental images; Second, *preoperational* (2–7 years), use of language or play as mental presentations; Third, *concrete* (7–11 years), concepts of weight, length, rules; Fourth, *formal operations* (11–15 years), reason using verbal propositions, hypotheses, and abstractions. (*APA 100–101. CTP 256–62. Har 611.*)

10. **(3)** Piaget's third stage of cognitive development is called *concrete operations*. See discussion in questions 9 and 11. (*APA 100–101. Har 611. CTP 256–62.*)

11. **(4)** Piaget's second major stage of cognitive or intellectual development is called *preoperational* (see question 9), which includes deferred imitation, symbolic play, graphic imagery (drawings), mental imagery, and language. (*CTP 258, 260. Har 611.*) Other developments in Piaget's four stages are as follows:

    First. *Sensorimotor*, which has six substages: (1) inborn motor and sensory reflexes, (2) primary circular reaction and first habits, (3) secondary circulatory reaction, (4) use of familiar means to obtain ends, (5) tertiary circular reaction and discovery through active experimentation, and (6) insight and object permanence.

    Second. See questions 9 and 62.

Third. *Concrete operations*, conservation of quantity, volume, weight, length, and time, based on reversibility by inversion or reciprocity, operation; class inclusion and seriation.

Fourth. *Formal operations*, whereby variables are isolated and all possible combinations are examined; hypothetical-deductive thinking; relationships formed.

12. (2) In Winnicott's object relations theory, transitional objects represent a way station between hallucinatory omnipotence and the acceptance of objective reality. A blanket or a toy (the object) helps the child negotiate the gradual shift from the experience of subjectivity to the sense of objectivity and can be considered a substitute for the mother's breast. (*CTP 382. Har 188.*)

13. (2) Gender identity develops early in life, is generally established by age 3, and depends on the sex in which an individual is reared regardless of biological factors. Once firmly established, it is extremely resistant to change. (*CTP 365, 1063. Har 588.*)

14. (3) A poor fit between a child's temperament and the parent's expectations leads to many psychological problems. However, there is no specific correlation with later specific behavior problems. Temperament by some definitions is the "reflecting nature" or internal behavior patterns learned from the culture, upbringing, and the internalization of relationships and social mores. It also refers to a behavioral style, presents as a measurement problem, is not immutable, and is difficult to identify by stable measures across time. (*CTP 554, 1355, 1692.*)

15. (4) The *anal phase* of psychosocial development (age 1½–3 years) is concerned with a sense of power over the environment and a consolidation of individual separation. There are emotional object constancy and development and integration of the ego with internalization of parents' demands and development of superego precursors. (*CTP 364. Har 175.*)

16. (3) According to Erikson, *integrity versus despair* is the eighth phase of psychosocial conflict of late life. Integrity is the acceptance of one's life as one's own responsibility. (*APA 96, 145. CTP 408. Har 668.*)

17. (4) The anal phase of psychosexual development is similar to Erikson's second phase of developmental tasks, autonomy versus shame. Erikson's industry versus inferiority is similar to latency; initiative versus guilt, oedipal; intimacy versus isolation, young adult; integrity versus despair, maturity. (*APA 96, 145. CTP 405–6.*)

18. (2) According to Mahler, an emotionally secure 2- to 3-year-old child has reliable internal representation of mother, which affords comfort with her absence and facilitates the child's ability to engage in independent activity. (*APA 110, 111.*)

19. (1) Bowlby (1969) observed that there is a biological purpose of attachment, which provides emotional security and social autonomy for the child. He described three stages in the child's reaction to loss: protest, despair, and detachment. About two-thirds of 1-year-old children show mild protest on departure of mother and are easily placated by her on return: these infants are classified as "securely attached." Infants who do not protest or approach mother on return (about 25%) are classified as "avoidant" or detached. Resistant or anxiously attached infants (about 10%) become markedly upset (despair) by mother's departure and resist mother's effort to comfort them. (*APA 110. Har 609–10.*)

20. (2) Most mental retardation (85%) is mild and is not recognized until school age or in adolescence. The majority of mentally retarded have normal birth, head size, and physical characteristics. Only about 5% have severe forms of retardation requiring long-term institutionalization. (*APA 704–5. CTP 1748–50.*)

21. (1) Pica is the most common cause of lead poisoning. Lead poisoning is one of the most frequent causes of acute toxic encephalopathy in young children. Symptoms are vomiting, irritability and clumsiness, progressing to seizures, stupor, and coma. There is a 15% mortality rate, and 25% develop permanent morbidity problems. Treatment is with EDTA, calcium disodium edetate. Other heavy metals that may cause similar CNS problems are mercury, arsenic, and manganese. (*CTP 207, 1861.*)

22. (2) Elective mutism occurs in males and females, but most studies report that females have a two times greater frequency than males. It generally starts at ages 3 to 5 years, before starting school. There is no organic pathology by definition, as the child consciously refuses to speak. About 50% have immaturity of speech. These children are generally described as negativistic, shy, and withdrawn, with sadistic and aggressive behavior similar to that of a 2-year-old. Frequently there are associated urinary and bowel difficulties. Elective mutism must be differentiated from disuse of speech (schizophrenia), deafness, aphasia, and conversion reactions. (*CTP 1887–89. APA 694–97.*)

23. (2) Children who become burn patients generally show psychic numbing, are not amnestic, and have no flashbacks. However, these patients show post-traumatic play of the reenactment of the event, and have a limited view of future. In general, burn patients show a high incidence of alcohol and other substance abuse, and accident proneness. Initially after discharge, all patients show anxiety, depression, and phobic behavior: these

symptoms are likely to be more marked with children. Burn patients with good premorbid personalities show better recovery over the first year. (*CTP 1233, 1276. Har 408.*)

24. (2) Enuresis can be treated with low nighttime doses of the tricyclic imipramine, 25 mg for those under age 12, 50–75 mg and up to 100 mg after age 12. Effects can be seen within one week, with one-third becoming non-enuretic and two-thirds having decreased wetting. Long-term success is poor with only 15% dry after discontinuance of drug: most relapse after three months. The reason for the tricyclic anti-enuretic effect is not known, but it is not due to the anticholinergic property. Common side effects of imipramine when it is used for treating children with enuresis are nervousness, sleep disorders, tiredness, and mild gastrointestinal disturbances. Treatment of enuresis with mechanical devices shows an initial 80% success rate, but 40% relapse after stopping treatment. Psychotherapy is not generally indicated unless there is other underlying psychopathology. (*APA 690–92. CTP 1882, 1938.*)

25. (2) There is a 20–60% incidence of ADHD in Tourette's disorder. Hyperactivity decreases or is better controlled in adolescence, but learning deficits and cognitive problems continue. Symptoms usually start in preschool years, but ADHD is usually not diagnosed until after entry into elementary school. Usually IQ is in the normal range. (*CTP 1831–32. APA 656.*)

26. (3) Kubler-Ross described five stages of dying seen after 7–13 years of age: (1) shock and denial; (2) anger; (3) bargaining; (4) depression; and (5) acceptance. These stages neither have to occur in sequence nor do patients necessarily go through each stage. (*CTP 1340–41. Har 729.*)

27. (4) *Fetal alcohol syndrome* is characterized by mental retardation, short stature, microcephaly, short palpebral fissures, mid-facial hypoplasia, plus possible cardiac defects or fine-motor dysfunctions. Low birth weight and developmental defects can increase incidence of infant mortality. (*CTP 1743. APA 317.*)

28. (3) Severe mental retardation is associated with inborn errors of metabolism, the majority related to autosomal recessive genes. Occasionally there are single gene or chromosomal aberrations, or polygenic familial syndromes as a cause. Previously, 3% of the retarded population was considered severely retarded, but some studies now state the figure is 1%. (*CTP 1729, 1739.*) The breakdown of the retarded population is as follows:

Category	IQ Range	% of Retarded Population
Mild	50–55 to 70	85%
Moderate	35–40 to 50–55	10%
Severe	20–25 to 35–40	3–4%
Profound	< 20–25	1–2%

29. (4) Major side effects of psychostimulants (sympathomimetics) are appetite suppression, insomnia, headaches, stomachaches, irritability, growth reduction, and tics. Insomnia, loss of appetite, and irritability usually disappear in four weeks. After 6–8 years of use, about 5–10 pounds decrease and 1/2″–1″ reduction in predicted weight-height have been reported. (*APA 660–63. CTP 1836.*)

30. (4) *Fragile X syndrome* consists of mental retardation, craniofacial features of long ears and a long narrow face, short stature, pectus excavatum, and enlarged testicular volume at puberty. (*CTP 1741–42. APA 708.*)

31. (2) *Reactive attachment disorder* is manifested by marked disturbance in social relatedness occurring before 5 years of age, caused by grossly pathogenic care by the child's primary caregivers. (*CTP 1894. APA 697–98.*)

32. (3) Children at risk for abuse are those under 3 years old, with physical and mental disabilities or developmental delays. Women tend to perpetrate more physical abuse, whereas males are responsible for the majority of sexual abuse. Parents who abuse their children tend to have poor impulse control, poor relations with their spouse, depression and low self-esteem, and often were abused by their parents. It is common for abusing fathers to batter their wives, and for mothers to be overdependent. Alcohol abuse is a common factor in these families. (*CTP 1962–64. Har 631.*)

33. (3) The majority of sexually abused children are females under the age of 6 who have been repeatedly sexually abused by a known male (two-thirds of cases). Long-term sequelae are mistrust, poor self-image, depression, hysterical character traits, social withdrawal and impaired peer relations, poor school performance and cognitive impairments, substance abuse, delayed post-traumatic stress disorder (PTSD), increased sexual arousal, sexual avoidance, and inhibition. (*APA 573. CTP 1966–70. Har 630.*)

34. (2) Play is an integral component of psychotherapy and diagnostic interviewing of the child. It is a natural medium through which thoughts, feelings, conflicts, and fears can be communicated as well as a means of therapeutic intervention. The child's phase of development plays a major role in determining the type of therapeutic play technique used. (*CTP 1911–13. Har 614.*)

35. (2) In a 30-year follow-up study, Robins (1966) reviewed 500 children diagnosed with childhood antisocial behavior at a outpatient clinic. Higher incidence of physical injuries, illness, hospitalizations, and emergency room visits were found to be predictors of greater adult psychopathology. Those children with early onset, poor grades, and low socioeconomic status had poorer outcome, whereas those with greater socialization skills had a better prognosis. From this study, it was concluded that antisocial behavior in childhood predicted maladjustment and severe psychopathology, which occurred in 37% as adults. (APA 667–68.)

36. (4) Nightmares in childhood can occur at any age and may persist into adulthood. The child vividly recalls the dreams and is oriented on awakening, which is different from night terrors. Nightmares occur during REM sleep, generally in the second half of night. *Pavor nocturnus,* also called night/sleep terrors (incubus in adults), occurs in 1–4% of all children. It is more common in males, occurs mostly in 4–12-year-olds, and disappears during adolescence. However, it may begin in the second or third decade of life, but rarely after 40. It occurs during sleep stages 3/4, deep NREM, and is related to sleepwalking. It happens during the first half of night. The individual sits up, is agitated and frightened, and shows automatism, mydriasis, respiration, and tachypnea, but rarely remembers the phenomenon the next morning. Night terrors are a hyperarousal state. (CTP 1121–22. Har 166.)

37. (4) *Dream anxiety disorder,* nightmare, is common; the child remembers the dream. Sleep terror disorder is an arousal phenomenon, not a dream, and it is not remembered. (CTP 1121–22. Har 166.)

38. (5) Nightmares and night terrors commonly occur during school age and are dysfunctions associated with sleep (parasomnias), but are two different phenomena. Night terrors are associated with sleepwalking as child. (Refer to question 36 for more details.) (CTP 1121–22. Har 166.)

39. (4) Night terrors are more common in males, and as noted in question 36, do not occur in REM sleep, but appear during deep NREM sleep, stages 3/4. (CTP 1122. Har 166.)

40. (5) During puberty and early adolescence, girls mature several years earlier than boys and are initially taller than boys. Boys eventually catch up and exceed the girls' height. (Har 642–44.)

41. (4) By age 2 or 3 years, almost all children have a firm conviction that they are male or female. Between 3 and 5 years, the concept of a private self that is not seen by others begins to be elaborated. By age 6 years, children accept that they cannot change into an animal or the opposite sex, and they begin to expand relations with peers and teachers. (APA 112. CTP 362–63.)

42. (3) Anorexia nervosa usually is seen in adolescent or young adult females (95% of cases), who are more than 15% under expected weight, have amenorrheas and problems with food, and abuse laxatives. If a DST is performed, it is generally abnormal. These patients show a fear of obesity and a disturbance of body image. (CTP 874, 1854–64. APA 265, 755–59.)

43. (2) Anorexia patients are more likely to exercise excessively (ballet, dancing, jogging). Binge eating, use of laxatives and diuretics, and vomiting can cause a metabolic change that may result in cardiac failure. Family, genetic, and endocrine studies have demonstrated associations among eating disorders, depression, and alcoholism. (APA 755–9. CTP 1854–64. Har 435–40.)

44. (1) Girls have a greater incidence of elective mutism than do boys, whereas boys have a greater incidence than do girls of stuttering, ADHD, mild mental retardation, and Tourette's disorder. (APA 694–96.)

45. (3) Identity disorder, role confusion (Erikson), or acute identity diffusion generally occurs in late adolescence, and is usually resolved in the mid-20s. There is a clinical picture of increased anxiety, depression, regression (loss of interest in friends, school, or activities), irritability, sleep difficulty, change of eating habits, and confusion and ambivalence about long-standing goals (career, sexuality, religion, friends). There is also an inability to integrate aspects of the self-identity, which may result in a "negative identity" (Erikson). (CTP 1889–90. Har 646.)

46. (4) Custody of a child is based on legal procedure and is usually decided according to the best interest of child. (CTP 1409. APA 1082.)

47. (2) About 75% of autistic children are mentally retarded and have severe developmental disorders with an absence of hallucinations and delusions. Seizures often develop during adolescence. There is an increased incidence of autism in siblings and families with more male than female cases (4 or 5 to 1). (APA 711–19. CTP 1772–87.)

48. (2) *Developmental reading disorder* is manifested by spelling and writing difficulties but good math skills, and is not related to a decrease in intelligence. This syndrome occurs in 5–10% of school-age children, with a male to female ratio of 4:1. There is an association with conduct disorders, and juvenile delinquency (15–20%); these problems usually persist into adulthood. It is common to have other family members with similar

problems. Difficulty with right-left discrimination is seen but with minimal dyspraxia. Associated allergies are also common. (*APA 720–24. CTP 1788–90.*)

49. **(4)** Conduct disorders occur more commonly in boys with lower IQs and academic and social difficulties. Ten to 15% of child referrals to outpatient clinics are diagnosed as conduct disorders. Parents of children with conduct disorders are more likely to be antisocial or have problems with alcohol. These children have more accidents, injuries, and hospital visits, and have an increased incidence of EEG abnormalities, epilepsy, ADHD, and suicidal behavior. (*APA 664–70. CTP 1821–28. Har 618.*)

50. **(3)** Various surveys of high-school seniors show the following substance use patterns: alcohol is the most frequently used, followed by marijuana and cigarettes, and then by cocaine. Heroin is the least used. (*CTP 645.*)

51. **(A)** Lawrence Kohlberg described six stages in the scheme of moral development in childhood based on "cross-cultural universals." For example, increased babbling during the second half of the first year is seen in all cultures, and occurs in the third or fourth stage of his six stages. (*CTP 293, 1357.*)

52. **(A)** Rene Spitz (1965) derived from direct observation of infants his "genetic field theory" of three organizers based on a embryological model. The first organizer is the "smiling response," which occurs around 6 weeks, and is a consistent repeatable social smile in response to a full face. The second organizer is the "stranger response," which occurs at 7 months, where the child turns away from a stranger with apprehension, anxiety. The third organizer is the development of the signal for "NO," which occurs in the toddler, 12–16 months, representing separation from mother. *Shame* is an emotion resulting from the failure to live up to self-expectation, (superego) guilt. (*APA 96–97, 100–101, 109.*)

53. **(B)** *Concrete operational thinking* is the third stage of Piagetian cognitive development: first is sensory-motor, second is preoperational, and fourth is formal operations. (*APA 96–97, 100–101.*)
    Conscience is commonly equated with the superego, whereas *conscious* is content of mind or mental functioning of which one is aware, awake, and alert. (Refer to question 52 and the third organizer of "no" response.)

54. **(D)** Separation anxiety is a normal development milestone and occurs by 10 months of age. The child follows or protests when mother leaves. According to Otto Rank and Freud, separation anxiety becomes heir to primal birth anxiety. Separation anxiety is also Spitz's second organizer, occurring at 7 months. (See question 52.) (*APA 96, 110, 155.*)

55. **(D)** Attachment research has shown that, when mother leaves and returns, young children (12–18 months) respond as follows: two-thirds, who are securely attached, show mild protest and are easily placated on return, one-fourth are classified as avoidant as they do not protest and do not approach mother, and 10%, who are resistant or anxiously attached, become markedly upset and resist efforts to be comforted. (*APA 97, 110. Har 614–15.*)

56. **(C)** *Stranger anxiety* starts at about 7 months (Spitz), is developed by 10 months and marks the attachment to familiar others, but fear of strangers. It is also called 7-month wariness by Gesell, who described expressions of wariness and fear in presence of a stranger. (*APA 96–97, 109.*) Questions 57, 58, 59, 63, and 64 are summarized in the chart on page 17.

57. **(C)** Refer to landmarks of normal development for a 2-month-old infant. (*APA 97–99.*)

58. **(B)** Refer to landmarks of normal development for a 1-year-old child. (*APA 97–99. CTP 1702.*)

59. **(C)** Refer to landmarks of normal development for a 3-year-old child. (*APA 100, 105. CTP 1702.*)

60. **(C)** Mahler described *object constancy* as beginning at 24–30 months. Object constancy marks the beginning of developing independence and separation from mother. (*APA 147. CTP 363–64.*)

61. **(A)** Rapprochement is a normal phase of development where the 2-year-old child has mixed feelings about a growing awareness and enjoyment of being separate coupled with a wish for closeness to mother in particular and a wish for her reassurance. (*APA 146–47. Har 609.*)

62. **(B)** Piaget's second major stage of cognitive development, the preoperational stage, consists of the appearance of symbolic functions and the beginning of internalized actions (ages 2–3 1/2 years), representational organization based on static configurations (4–5 1/2 years), and detailed representational regulation (5 1/2–7 years). (*APA 100–101. CTP 256–62. Har 611.*)

63. **(C)** Refer to landmarks of normal development for a 2-year-old child. (*APA 99. CTP 1702.*)

64. **(B)** One way of remembering and describing children's development levels is to THINK "SMALL"; S—social (psychosocial), M—motor (neuromuscular), A—adaptive, LL—learning and language. (*APA 99. CTP 1702.*) (See table next page)

65. **(A)** Winnicott suggested that one cannot conceptually understand a baby's development without considering

LANDMARKS OF NORMAL DEVELOPMENT (Based on Gesell)

Age	Social	Motor	Adaptive	Language
2 mos.	Follows a moving person, smiles	Symmetric posture, head erect with bobbing	Follows an object past midline	Sustained "cooing" and vocalizes in response to social interaction
1 year	Points, hugs, and offers toy	Walks several steps, turns pages	Imitates scribbles, puts round blocks in formboard, releases toy	Six words, uses jargon
18 mos.	Gets spoon to mouth correctly, hands empty dish, echoes two or more last words, imitates parents' activities (i.e., work)	Walks down stairs with one hand held, builds tower of two to four blocks	Imitates stroke of crayon, places three blocks in formboard	20-29 words plus names of sibs, friends, relatives, combines two to three words, asks for more food and drink
2 years	Helps put things away, calls self or "me," occasionally indicates toilet needs	Jumps, both feet off floor, kicks large ball, builds tower out of blocks	Imitates vertical stroke and circular scribble, inserts circle, triangle in formboard	50 plus words, three- to four-word sentences, uses "I" and "you," uses plurals
3 years	Toilet trained, takes turns, plays with other children, washes and dries hands	Alternates feet going downstairs, throws ball overhand, builds tower of ten blocks	Copies vertical and horizontal strokes, circle, imitates cross, repeats three digits	Recites a song, knows up and down, and or but, follows three commands on under, beside, in back and in front of, knows two colors

the role of mother. He stated that a "good enough" mother will respond to a child's communication and meet its needs adequately, though not perfectly. He postulated an intermediate stage of separation-individuation where the infant relates to transitional objects. (*APA 141. CTP 382. Har 188.*)

66. **(D)** The child at 1 1/2 to 4 years is physiologically and psychologically ready for toilet training. A combination of mild disapproval of wetting and social rewards for self-control and appropriate toilet use appears to work best. Early coercive toilet training does not lead to enuresis or encopresis but may produce other emotional disturbances. (*CTP 1879–80.*)

67. **(D)** *Gender identity* is the psychological experience of the self as a male or female, masculine or feminine. Gender role is the behavioral aspect of socially acting as a male or female. It is consolidated and developed by age 3 to 5 years. Biology, individual psychology, and socialization interact to form and evolve the components of sexual identity. (*CTP 1061–64.*)

68. **(E)** S. Chess and A. Thomas identified nine behavioral differences in temperament and autonomic activity: (1) spontaneous "activity level," threshold, intensity, and duration of reactions to external stimuli; (2) regularity or irregularity of certain biological "rhythms" such as sleep, hunger, elimination; (3) tendencies to "approach or withdraw" from new stimuli and adaption to them, such as new food, toy, or person; (4) the speed and ease of "adaptability to altered environmental structuring"; (5) "intensity reaction" and energy used in mood expression; (6) "threshold of responsiveness" to sensory stimuli, environment, social contacts; (7) "quality of mood" from pleasant to unpleasant; (8) "distractibility" from environmental stimuli interfering with or altering direction of behavior; and (9) "attention span and persistence" to pursue and maintain activity. (*CTP 554.*)

69. **(D)** Three categories of infant temperament were described by Thomas, Chess, and Birch (1968), as easy, slow to warm up, and difficult. (*CTP 554. Har 626.*)

70. **(A)** Refer to question 15 for explanation of the anal phase of development. In addition, there are struggles for cleanliness and orderliness; issues of stubbornness, defiance, and ambivalence; and feelings of omnipotence. (*CTP 364. Har 175.*)

71. **(D)** The oral phase of development is divided into three phases: (1) attachments; (2) trusting and affectionate relationships; (3) sucking and biting. During the oral phase there is the development of object constancy and relationship with the mother. (*CTP 363. Har 174–75.*)

72. **(A)** The Oedipus complex in boys is less complicated than for girls because the boy remains attached to his first love object, the mother. It occurs during ages 3 to 5 years and is the climax of development and of infantile sexuality. Gender identity becomes consolidated as significance of anatomical sexual differences is understood. Problems in resolution predispose to adult psychoneurosis. In males, even though the Oedipus complex is resolved at age 5 or 6, it can be reactivated in the form of castration complex during puberty. (*CTP 364–65. Har 175–76.*)

73. **(B)** Females, during the oedipal period, must shift their primary attachment from mother to father. The phase is resolved when the father does not comply with daughter's sexual wishes and mother disapproves of the wishes toward father. The resolution of the feminine Oedipus complex leads to feminine superego and normal psychosexual development. (*CTP 364–65, 374. Har 176.*)

74. **(A)** Inadequate care can be on the level of physical and/or emotional abuse and can cause long-term behavioral changes, hyperactivity, short stature, and lowered IQ. The hallmarks of chronic abuse are grossly disturbed interpersonal relationships and retardation of body growth. (*APA 697–99. Har 626. CTP 1898–99.*)

75. **(C)** *Intimacy versus isolation* is stage 6 of Erik Erikson's (1963) "epigenetic" eight phases of psychosocial crisis in development, which cover the entire life span. The stages are as follows:

    Stage 1. *Basic trust versus basic mistrust* (similar to oral-sensory, birth to 2 years); the stage of acquisition of sense that the universe is reliable and that our most important object relations are consistent and available.

    Stage 2. *Autonomy versus shame and doubt* (muscular-anal, 2–4 years); the attainment of control of body functions and mobility and thinking. There is now a concern about disappointment in oneself and important figures.

    Stage 3. *Initiative versus guilt* (similar to Freud and Abraham's oedipal, phallic-locomotor, 4–7 years); ideal prototypes are developed.

    Stage 4. *Industry versus inferiority* (latency, 7 years to adolescence); language and learning are developed.

    Stage 5. *Identity versus role confusion* (puberty and adolescence); the clarification of issues of personal identity and the depersonification of internal representations.

    Stage 6. *Intimacy versus isolation* (young adult, early mature adulthood); rediscovering attachments and mature bonding.

    Stage 7. *Generactivity versus stagnation*; creative productive adulthood.

    Stage 8. *Ego integrity versus despair*; maturity, later adulthood, vital involvement. This may be two stages, time of retirement up to age 85, and age 85 to death. (*APA 145. CTP 405–9. Har 190, 613.*)

76. **(C)** Motor skills landmarks in a normal developing child:

    15 months—spontaneous scribble
    18 months—imitates stroke of crayon
    24 months—imitates vertical stroke, circular scribble
    30 months—imitates horizontal stroke, circle
    36 months—copies vertical and horizontal stroke, copies circle, imitates cross
    48 months—draws person with two parts
    60 months—adds eight parts to incomplete man, copies square (54 months) and triangle (*APA 99–100.*)

77. **(E)** See question 59 (p. 6) and chart (p. 17) referring to the 3-year-old's social, motor, adaptive, and language abilities. (*APA 100.*)

78. **(E)** In assessing suicide risk in a child or adolescent, it is important to evaluate various factors such as genetic vulnerability (history of suicidal behavior in families, depression, alcoholism, and other mental disorders), child's depression and suicidal ideation (how would the act be accomplished), the child's concept of death, alcohol or substance abuse by the child, physiological changes (e.g., sleep, eating, weight changes), separation from parents, and, also important, the parent's attitude. (*APA 1029–31. Har 621–22*)

79. **(D)** Teenage suicide is often associated with conduct disorders, hostility, aggression, and assaultiveness. Depression and use of alcohol and drugs are important factors. Suicide is the third leading cause of death in the 15- to 24-year-old age group, and the seventh leading cause of death in the 5- to 14-year-old age group. The rate peaks in early adulthood, then falls off until it increases in middle age to peak again in old age. (*APA 1029–31. Har 651–52.*)

IQ level	Mild 50-55 to 70	Moderate 35-40 to 50-55	Severe 20-25 to 40	Profound <20-25
% of MR pop:	85%	10%	4%	1%
Description:	educable	trainable	untrainable	untrainable
Grade level:	6th	2nd	<1st	
Placement:	community placement	sheltered workshop	structured environment	institutional placement

80. **(B)** A child's concept of death depends on age.

Age 3-5: it is reversible, similar to sleep, and due to violence, seen in concrete terms, temporary and personified

Age 5: recognizes not immune to accidents

Age 5-7: it is externally caused, a fact of life, and inevitable

Age 6-9: it becomes more personified, and it is definitely understood to be irreversible

Age 8-12: a universal fact, similar to adults (*Har 738-43. CTP 1340.*)

81. **(A)** Down's syndrome, caused by a trisomy 21 and also a rarer form of abnormal chromosome 15 containing fragment from 21, may be manifested by progressive neuropathological changes similar to Alzheimer's disease, and with congenital heart defects. (*Har 139, 370. CTP 1739-41. APA 708.*)

82. **(B)** Down's syndrome patients are likely to have hearing problems (70%), increased incidence of hypothyroidism (20% by age 30-40) and seizures (5-10%), ocular difficulties, hypotonia, congenital heart disorders (1/3), and gastrointestinal anomalies (1/10). Most Down's syndrome patients are in the "trainable" category (IQ 35-55, moderate to severe), are able to achieve 2nd grade status, and do not need institutional care. (*CTP 1739-41. Har 685.*)

83. **(C)** The prevalence of severe mental retardation is 1-3%, with the ratio of males to females being 1.5-3:1. The table on this page delineates the classification and level of adjustments that may be expected at various IQ levels. (*APA 704-5. Har 682-83.*)

84. **(B)** Mentally retarded individuals are at a 2-4 times risk of developing emotional disorders. Fifty percent have additional mental disorder diagnoses. About one-half to one-third have ADHD symptoms. The reported diagnosis of mental retardation is low at preschool age years, increases in early school years, peaks in late school years (age 15), and then declines during adulthood (1%). (*APA 704-6. CTP 1748-50.*)

85. **(A)** In addition to substance use and abuse (alcohol, cocaine, certain medications), the incidence of mental retardation is increased by maternal infections (rubella, toxoplasmosis, syphilis), toxic exposure (alcohol, lead poisoning, anticonvulsants, radiation), malnutrition, kernicterus, trauma, illnesses (toxemia, diabetes, hypoglycemia), and genetic defect (trisomy 21, sex chromosome abnormalities). (*APA 707. CTP 1742-46. Har 686-87.*)

86. **(E)** The most common methods of preventing mental retardation, in addition to providing good prenatal care and prevention of those conditions listed in question 85, are by treating infants with cretinism (thyroid medication), lead intoxication (EDTA and dimercaprol [BAL]), phenylketonuria (PKU) (dietary elimination of phenylalanine), and Wilson's disease (eliminate copper from body with penicillamine, trientine HCl). (*CTP 1740-41. Har 685-86.*)

87. **(E)** *Pica* is the repeated ingestion of nonnutritive substances such as clay, plaster, dirt, and paper. Anywhere from 10-30% of children between 1 and 6 years and about 10-20% of people at some point in life have pica. Pica is increased with mental retardation; pregnant females in certain cultures and low socioeconomic states eat starch and clay. Problems created by pica are constipation, GI malabsorption and the resulting anemias, traumatic intestinal bleeding, fecal impactions, obstructions, salt imbalances, parasitic infections, vomiting, accidental poisonings, and lead encephalopathy. These can produce slow motor and mental development, neurological deficits, and behavioral abnormalities in the child. (*APA 679-81. CTP 1854, 1857, 1861.*)

88. **(E)** A blind child who has physical findings of normal pupillary reactions and optic fundi (e.g., cortical blindness) may be mistaken as having psychogenic blindness. The blind child's lack of facial expression may incorrectly be perceived as la belle indifference while the tendency of the blind child to touch and feel may be anxiety arousing. (*CTP 239, 606t.*)

89. **(C)** Diabetes mellitus, a chronic illness, can result in lowered self-image, feelings of loss, grief, fear, helplessness, and shame or guilt. (*Har 622-23. CTP 1288-89.*)

90. **(E)** About 2-5% of children in grade school have a stuttering disorder lasting typically for two to four years. Fifty to 80% have a spontaneous improvement. About 5% persist into adolescence. About 1% of ado-

lescents and adults have this problem. There is a male to female ratio of 3–4:1. Theories of etiology range from genetic (20–40% within families), neurological, psychodynamic, and behavioral concepts, but precise mechanisms are not known. (*APA 693. CTP 579, 1810–12.*)

91. **(C)** Functional enuresis occurs in 25% of boys under the age of 5 years. Between age 5 and age 10 years, 5–7% of boys and 3% of girls are enuretic, and after age 10 years, 3% of boys and 2% of girls. There is a 1% prevalence rate in adults. Seventy percent of enuretics have first-degree relatives with similar problem. About one-half have smaller bladders, small volume on voiding, and other physical findings such as short stature and low mean bone age. Some reports indicate that there is delayed sexual development in adolescence. (*APA 690–92. CTP 1879–82.*)

92. **(C)** Predictors of bipolar outcome in adolescents and young adults indicate a better prognosis if there is acute onset with major manic signs and symptoms, but a worse outcome with major depression or mixed symptomatology. Other factors predicting future bipolar disorders are acute onset, hypersomnic, retarded or psychotic depression, postpartum onset, tricyclic hypomania, bipolar family history, loaded pedigree, and family history of mood disorder in consecutive generations. (*CTP 1991. APA 413. Har 322–23.*)

93. **(A)** Depression and conduct disorder, especially aggressive type, are common factors in teenage suicide. Months prior to the suicidal behavior, 40% have been reported to have been drunk at least three times per week, and 40–50% were involved with aggressive antisocial behavior. Depression and aggressive symptoms coexist more often in adolescents than in adults. (*CTP 1992. Har 659.*)

94. **(B)** Depressed affect in children is most often accompanied by low self-esteem: "I can't do that," "I'm no good." These children often show fatigue, loss of interest and pleasure, guilt, difficulty in concentrating (especially at school), and disturbance in sleep and motor activity. In addition, the clinician must ask about suicidal fantasies and actions. Child or parental depression and suicide checklists may be used as an adjunct to patient interview. Adults, parents, and teachers tend to underestimate child and adolescent depression. (*CTP 1724–25, 1716. APA 168. Har 620–21.*)

95. **(C)** In addition to death being seen as reversible, a disappearance, and immobility by a 4-year-old, children of this age are also dealing with separation anxiety and struggling for autonomy; these are factors that can complicate a child's reaction to a death. (See question 80.) (*CTP 1340. Har 738–43.*)

96. **(C)** See question 30 discussing the Fragile X syndrome, and question 27 for the fetal alcohol syndrome. (*CTP 204, 1743. APA 317.*)

97. **(C)** Phenylketonuria (PKU) is an inborn error of metabolism, and is associated with eczema, blonde hair, musty odor, and mental retardation. (*CTP 1741. Har 139.*)

98. **(C)** Treatment of ADHD is with tricyclics (imipramine, desipramine) and psychostimulants. Tolerance to medications, especially the tricyclics, can develop over time. Imipramine can cause confusion and agitation. Very little learning improvement is seen with medications in children with severe LD and ADHD. There may be a degree of improvement when medications are used with some specific LD's. (*CTP 1831–35. APA 990–94. Har 618.*)

99. **(E)** Children with ADHD usually have problems with peers because of their behavior. Siblings have a five to six times greater incidence of ADHD. (*CTP 1828–37.*)

100. **(E)** In addition to question 99, there is an increased incidence of alcoholism, antisocial personality, and Briquet's syndrome (somatization) in relatives, especially females. Hyperactivity may be less during a one-to-one interaction or in a nondistracting (more structured, low stimulus) environment. (*CTP 1828–37.*)

101. **(D)** Psychostimulants may or may not help children with learning disabilities, depending on what type of learning problems are present. Once off medications, previous behavior problems can reoccur. (Refer to question 98.) (*APA 990–94. CTP 1831–35.*)

102. **(D)** Medications for ADHD (particularly methylphenidate), in decreasing order of effectiveness (*CTP 1835–36. APA 660–63*):
    1) improve impulse control and enhance reflection
    2) decrease restlessness and fidgetiness
    3) improve social skills and interaction
    4) cognitive organization more efficient
    5) improve fine motor coordination

103. **(E)** The recommended doses of imipramine for children with enuresis, ADHD, depressive disorders, and school phobia are 1–2 mg/kg, with maximum of 5 mg/kg. The drug can lower seizure threshold, causes increased pulse rate and EKG changes, tremors, increased aggressiveness and temper outbursts. (Refer to question 98 regarding tolerance.) (*CTP 1936.*)

104. **(E)** Abused children are more likely to suffer from cognitive and developmental impairments and difficulties in school adjustment. Pathological object relationships, primitive defense mechanisms (denial, projection, splitting), poor self-concept, sadness and depres-

sion, caution, and pseudomaturity can often persist. Impaired impulse control and CNS impairments (organic mental change) due to increased physical injuries, post-traumatic stress disorder (PTSD), and masochistic and self-destructive behavior are also common problems seen later in life. (*CTP 1964–65. Har 631.*)

105. (E) Because child abuse is both a medical and legal problem, some courts are allowing videotapes to be submitted in order to obtain data, to reduce the number of persons interviewing the child victim, and to spare the child the pain of facing the perpetrator in court. During an interview with a victim of sex abuse, the clinician should try to get the patient to describe details of the alleged abuse and identify the responsible person. The clinician should note the child's comments in the child's own words. If abuse is described or played out by the child, the abuse likely took place. Denial of the problem does not mean sex abuse did not occur. Protecting the child from further abuse is the first priority. The majority of perpetrators are male and someone known to the child or family. Almost all female sexual abusers are mentally ill. (*CTP 1966–69. Har 632.*)

106. (B) In comparing adult and child psychotherapy, transference is different with children, where it is less intense and of limited therapeutic usefulness. There are more verbal and behavior interactions utilizing learning theory when working with children. The therapist must be a more active force for change. Capacity for self-observation by the child patient is limited. Major goals are habilitative rather than rehabilitative, and the clinician must serve as the parent surrogate, teacher, and personal friend. (*CTP 1910–13. Har 450–51, 615–16. APA 1002–3.*)

107. (D) In the psychotherapy of children and adolescents, it is essential to consider their environment and family dynamics and to work with agencies such as schools and courts. Optimally, parents should be part of a therapeutic alliance. (*CTP 1914–18. APA 1002–3.*) The basic tenets of child psychoanalysis are as follows:

1) defenses are interpreted before drives
2) surfaced conscious material is interpreted first
3) external influences are considered in making interpretations
4) interpretations of the patient conflicts are offered to allow the patient to develop a balanced picture of self
5) analyst talks and relates to patient in an empathic manner taking into account patient affect

Psychoanalytic psychotherapy has four basic tenets:

1) unconscious mental functions are important
2) manifest behavior is based on internalized conflicts
3) symptoms have a psychological meaning to the child

4) transference provides an understanding of the child-therapist relationship based on prior experiences with parent and significant others

Goals are teaching, clarifying, interpreting, and healing, as well as comforting through alliance formation. Family-parental participation in treatment is essential. The role of play is to help with clarification, reassurance, suggestion, abreaction, manipulation, and to provide for corrective emotional experience and interpretation. Termination takes place when presenting problems are resolved and in as constructive a manner as possible.

108. (A) Refer to questions 98 and 103. Imipramine has a therapeutic window. (*CTP 1934–40. APA 990–94. Har 618.*)

109. (C) A study of autistic children revealed that haloperidol, 2–10 mg/day, may be helpful for promoting learning, controlling behavior symptoms (reduction of withdrawal), reducing excessive activity levels and enhancing the effect of behavior therapies (more effective active and imitative speech). The use of haloperidol with behavior therapy was more effective than either used alone. The major adverse effect is excessive sedation, which is dose-related. Haloperidol is most helpful with autistic patients who are hyperactive or normoactive, disruptive, or showing temper tantrums, but it is not helpful with those who are anergic or hypoactive. (*CTP 1785–86, 1936–37. APA 716.*)

110. (C) Reported indications for using antipsychotics with children are schizophrenia, severe uncontrolled aggressive conduct disorder, autistic disorder, Tourette's disorder, and mental retardation with severe aggression to self or others. (*CTP 1936–38.*) Untoward effects are drowsiness, extrapyramidal reactions (acute dystonic, akathisia, parkinsonian reaction, rabbit syndrome), tardive and withdrawal dyskinesia (seen as early as 2 months), elevated liver enzymes, weight gain, gynecomastia, amenorrhea, and galactorrhea.

111. (A) Children with oppositional defiant disorder manifest similar behavior normally seen in 18–36-month-old children. Negativism, hostility, and defiance are the usual symptoms typically shown in familiar settings, home, school, leisure-time activity, and with parents and other adults with whom the child has more contact. Commonly associated are ADHD, academic difficulties and, at a later age, substance abuse. The child may become the adult with passive aggressive personality disorder. (*CTP 1843–45. APA 670–72.*)

112. (E) One of the most effective treatments for obsessive compulsive disorders is the drug clomipramine (Anafranil), a tricyclic (tertiary amine) antidepressant. Its effectiveness may be due to its effects on serotonin neu-

ronal transmission. Recently, fluoxetine (Prozac), a potent uptake inhibitor of serotonin, has been found to have therapeutic benefit. Phenelzine (Nardil), a MAOI, has also been of value. However, regardless of the drugs used, many patients relapse when the medication is discontinued. Therefore, other therapies need to be pursued. (*CTP 1465–66. APA 478–79. Har 244–45.*) Psychotherapies to treat OCD include behavior therapies (grading and flooding techniques [see questions 10 and 11 in Chapter 5]), family therapy (see question 17 in Chapter 5), and analytic oriented psychotherapy (see questions 3, 4, and 20, Chapter 5).

113. **(C)** Imaginary companions most often appear during preschool years in 50% of children ages 3–10 years, and usually disappear around age 12. Imaginary companions help decrease anxiety. (*CTP 1708.*)

114. **(D)** During the 1940s, Bowlby extended studies on attachment to the hospital setting. At that time, mothers were separated from their infants and had very limited visiting hours. In addition, T. Brazelton's studies showed normal attachment occurred during the first month of life. These studies of infant bonding and the importance of contacts between mother and child have caused hospitals to change their approach to care by allowing rooming-in and frequent parent-child contacts. (*Har 609–10.*)

115. **(D)** See previous questions concerning night terrors, number 36; enuresis, number 91; and imaginary companions, number 113. A 3-year-old with persistent head-banging (usual beginning 6–12 months) after one year should be referred for evaluation. About 15–20% of normal pediatric population may have a history of transient stereotypes. Children with pervasive developmental disorder are more likely to show severe and profound mental retardation. Stereotypes and habits include head-banging, body-rocking, eye-poking, self-biting, teeth-grinding, thumb-sucking, and breath-holding. (*APA 700. CTP 1121–22.*)

116. **(B)** Prolonged thumb-sucking can cause dental problems. Thumb-sucking is present in most infants. (*CTP 364–65. Har 175.*)

117. **(D)** Separation anxiety is normal at 12–36 months. This symptom can be considered a disorder after 4 years of age and tends to run in families. Children less than 6 years old showing separation anxiety usually improve spontaneously. Haloperidol in the treatment of Tourette's disorder reduces tics but may cause the development of a separation anxiety disorder. (*CTP 1848–49. APA 673–77.*)

118. **(E)** School absenteeism is common; 75% of adults admit to this behavior during childhood. It may be a manifestation of family or cultural attitude (up to 90% of students in inner city schools), separation (anxiety disorder), conduct disorder (truancy), depression, and other psychiatric disorders (schizophrenia, pervasive developmental disorder). (*APA 674–75.*)

119. **(A)** Separation anxiety in grade school is a child psychiatric emergency and warrants prompt attention. Physical symptoms and signs of anxiety are likely to occur on Sundays and school days when the child fears separation from the parents. (See question 117 for more information.) (*APA 673–77. CTP 1847–49.*)

120. **(E)** Treatment of separation anxiety and school absenteeism must include the child (psychotherapy), parents (family therapy), peers (group support), and school. Early return to school is important. Academic problems must be identified and corrected. Medication may be necessary. (*CTP 1847–49. APA 673–77.*)

121. **(A)** Tourette's disorder prevalence is reported as being equal in males and females or in a ratio up to 3:1, male to female. It is more common in children with ADHD. Increased family history of tics and a greater risk of Tourette's disorder in relatives of female patients are reported. About 91% at age of onset are less than 11 years old and 99% by 15 years, with a typical age of onset 5–10 years old. (*APA 686–88. CTP 1869–70. Har 123.*)

122. **(E)** Tourette's disorder is a lifelong problem. Symptoms wax and wane in 97% of patients. Location of tics varies in 96%. In the basal ganglia dopamine system, there is either hyperactivity of dopamine neurons in the striatum or supersensitivity of postsynaptic receptors. Treatment is by using neuroleptics to block the dopamine type 2 (D2) receptors (see question 123). (*APA 686–88. CTP 1872–78.*)

123. **(A)** As noted in question 122, blockage of dopamine by drugs such as haloperidol, clonidine, and pimozide provides the most effective symptomatic treatment. (*APA 686–88. CTP 1872–78.*)

124. **(B)** Overanxious disorder in children presents with similar symptoms as in adults and tends to occur in families. Treatment includes diphenhydramine, benzodiazepines, and hydroxyzine. (*APA 677–79. CTP 1849–50.*)

125. **(E)** The prominent feature of borderline personality disorder is instability. In addition, these patients show eating disorders, functional encopresis, substance abuse, aggression, unpredictability, impulsivity, suicide attempts, antisocial behavior, and family conflicts. Genetically there is increased family history of mood disorders and ADHD. (*CTP 1891. APA 636–37. Har 347–49.*)

126. **(E)** Autistic symptoms are associated with retardation (75%), medical conditions such as PKU, encephalitis, and seizures (25% temporal lobe epilepsy–late childhood onset, and grand mal), massive infantile spasms (common, early onset), and Fragile X syndrome. (*APA 711–17. CTP 1772–84.*)

127. **(E)** Characteristics of infantile autism are: lack of awareness or feelings for others, lack of interest in people, and lack of seeking of comfort when anxious or in pain; abnormal and narrow preoccupations such as with parts of objects, spinning wheels; poor communications, such as echolalia, abnormal speech; no eye-to-eye contact, gaze avoidance, body movement stereotypes and overactivity, impaired imitation, abnormal social play, and poor peer relations. (*CTP 1779–1782. APA 711–7. Har 619.*)

128. **(B)** Autism is distributed evenly among socioeconomic classes. The cause is unknown. Treatment with low-dose haloperidol has been helpful (see question 109). The best prognosis is if the child has good nonverbal intelligence and useful speech by age 5. (*CTP 1779. APA 711–17. Har 619.*)

129. **(D)** Anaclitic depression was initially described by Spitz as usually occurring during the second to sixth month of life, but can occur even later (also called "Hospitalism" by Bowlby). It is developed after separation from mother and other caretakers, and in the extreme form results in marasmus and death. (*CTP 890, 1981–82. Har 325.*)

130. **(A)** Imaginary playmates are normal hallucinations and are false sensory perceptions not associated with real external stimuli. *Hypnagogic phenomena* occur while falling asleep. *Lilliputian hallucination* is the seeing of a reduction in size or of miniature people. *Eidetic images* are visual memories of almost hallucinatory vividness, that may be based in fantasy, dream, or actual memory. (*CTP 474. APA 1251. Har 40.*)

2

SUBSTANCE ABUSE
Alcohol and Drug Abuse

DIRECTIONS: Select the best single response for each of the questions 1 through 14.

1. Abrupt drug withdrawal is likely to be life threatening in a patient addicted to:

   1. Cocaine
   2. Heroin
   3. Meprobamate
   4. Phencyclidine
   5. Diazepam

2. In treating opioid overdose, which of the following is effective?

   1. Methadone
   2. L-alpha-acetylmethadol (LAAM)
   3. Naloxone
   4. Buprenorphine
   5. Clonidine

3. You are treating a pregnant heroin addict who wants to be sure that her baby is not harmed. Your best management would be:
   1. Maintain the patient on high-dose methadone
   2. Maintain the patient on low-dose methadone
   3. Withdraw the patient from opioids using clonidine
   4. Withdraw the patient from heroin using methadone
   5. Stop all opioids and treat withdrawal symptoms

4. Symptoms of heroin withdrawal include all of the following except:

   1. Twitching movements in the legs
   2. Grand mal seizures
   3. Increased blood pressure
   4. Diarrhea
   5. Dilated pupils

5. Which of the following statements about the pentobarbital challenge test are correct?

   1. It indicates starting dose of phenobarbital for sedative detoxification
   2. It is used to differentiate organic from psychogenic amnesia
   3. An intravenous barbiturate is given to facilitate emotional abreaction

4. It is a useful therapeutic procedure with abdominal pain due to porphyria
   5. The procedure validates organicity with the Bender Gestalt test

6. Cocaine abuse is likely to produce symptoms similar to which of the following?

   1. Major depression
   2. Paranoid schizophrenia
   3. Obsessive compulsive disorder
   4. General anxiety disorder
   5. Moderate mental retardation

7. A characteristic manifestation of hallucinogen use is:

   1. Bruxism
   2. Agoraphobia
   3. Neologisms
   4. Synesthesia
   5. Anomie

8. The management of phencyclidine toxicity is likely to include all of the following except:

   1. Naloxone for respiratory depression
   2. Diazepam for seizures
   3. Propranolol for adrenergic crisis
   4. Haloperidol for disorganized, disruptive behavior
   5. Low-stimulus environment

9. A 16-year-old boy is brought for emergency evaluation after taking some of his mother's medication in order to get "high." He is flushed and his pupils are dilated and only poorly reactive. He complains of dry mouth. He is restless, confused at times, and may be having visual hallucinations. Which of the following medications is he likely to have taken?

   1. Phenelzine
   2. Disulfiram
   3. Propranolol
   4. Alprazolam
   5. Benztropine

10. Which of the following statements about alcohol-induced blackouts are correct?

1. Remote memory deficit
2. Immediate memory deficit
3. Short-term memory deficit
4. All of the above
5. Does not occur in non-alcoholics

11. Medical complications of chronic alcoholism include all of the following except:

   1. Cardiomyopathy
   2. Chronic pancreatitis
   3. Hepatolenticular degeneration
   4. Fetal growth retardation
   5. Testicular atrophy

12. All of the following statements about alcohol withdrawal delirium are correct except:

   1. Does not occur while still drinking
   2. Withdrawal seizures are most common 24 hours after withdrawal
   3. Delirium tremens has peak incidence four days after withdrawal
   4. May be precipitated by surgery
   5. Well-nourished patients should be given vitamins

13. All of the following are symptoms of alcohol withdrawal except:

   1. Coarse tremor of hands or tongue
   2. Generalized tonic-clonic seizures
   3. Abducent nerve paresis or paralysis
   4. Tachycardia, sweating, dilated pupils
   5. Clouding of consciousness

14. In the management of alcohol withdrawal delirium, the clinician may wish to use all of the following except:

   1. Chlordiazepoxide
   2. Chlorpromazine
   3. Thiamine
   4. Intravenous glucose
   5. Magnesium sulfate

DIRECTIONS: For questions 15 through 50, one or more of the alternatives given are correct. After you decide which choices are correct, record your answer according to the following.

(A) if alternatives 1, 2 and 3 only are correct.
(B) if alternatives 1 and 3 only are correct.
(C) if alternatives 2 and 4 only are correct.
(D) if alternative 4 only is correct.
(E) if all four alternatives are correct.

15. When a person taking a medication or abusing a drug develops tolerance, which of the following statements are valid?

1. The same dosage of the drug has reduced effect
2. Tolerance develops uniformly to all effects of the drug
3. Physical dependence tends to develop in parallel with tolerance
4. Withdrawal symptoms are less likely after tolerance has developed

16. Which of the following statements are correct about heroin abuse?

   1. The peak incidence is age 25 to 35
   2. It affects men three times as often as women
   3. The majority of heroin abusers are involved in maintenance programs
   4. Most heroin abusers eventually stop on their own

17. In the management of detoxified substance-abusing patients in a therapeutic community, poor prognosis is more likely with:

   1. Coexisting severe psychopathology
   2. Dropout before three months
   3. Continued alcohol use
   4. Adjunctive use of antidepressants

18. Which of the following statements are correct in the treatment of pregnant opioid addicts?

   1. High-dose methadone maintenance leads to low-risk neonatal withdrawal
   2. Opioid withdrawal may lead to miscarriage or fetal death
   3. Women using opioids tend to have easy, uncomplicated deliveries
   4. Many opioid dependent women seek treatment when they become pregnant

19. Withdrawal convulsions are likely to occur in patients who have used chronically which of the following drugs?

   1. Secobarbital
   2. Desipramine
   3. Lorazepam
   4. Phencyclidine

20. In adults with no prior history of seizure disorder, seizures may be caused by:

   1. Phencyclidine intoxication
   2. Cocaine intoxication
   3. Amphetamine intoxication
   4. Meperidine intoxication

21. Which of the following statements about daily, heavy marijuana users are correct?

   1. Decrease in tachycardia caused by marijuana
   2. Detectable in urine 2–3 weeks after stopping

3. Reduced mood elevation effect

4. Reduced need to continue marijuana use

22. Which of the following statements about U.S. enlisted men who became addicted to opioids in Vietnam are correct?

   1. Nearly 90% did not become addicted again within three years of return to the United States
   2. Relapse more common in older white soldiers
   3. Higher relapse rate in sons of alcoholic parents
   4. About 75% of soldiers who used heroin five or more times became drug dependent

23. Symptoms of opioid toxicity include which of the following?

   1. Leg muscle twitching
   2. Pulmonary edema
   3. Seizures
   4. Hypothermia

24. Which of the following medications can be used therapeutically in the rehabilitation of opioid dependent patients?

   1. Methadone
   2. Naltrexone
   3. Clonidine
   4. Levo-alpha-acetylmethadol

25. The duration and severity of withdrawal symptoms in sedative-anxiolytic abusers depend on:

   1. Duration of drug use
   2. Amount of drug used
   3. Rate of elimination of drug and metabolites
   4. Method of drug administration

26. When a patient has been taking heavy doses of barbiturates for an extended period, early symptoms of withdrawal are likely to include:

   1. Weakness
   2. Insomnia
   3. Anxiety
   4. Tremulousness

27. Which of the following statements about the symptoms of barbiturate withdrawal are correct?

   1. Develops more quickly with secobarbital than phenobarbital abusers
   2. Cardiovascular collapse may be fatal
   3. Abdominal discomfort, nausea, and vomiting
   4. Seizures generally precede delirium

28. Which of the following statements about diazepam-dependent patients are correct?

   1. Withdrawal symptoms become disabling within 24 hours of stopping

2. Low alcohol intake may precipitate overdose

3. Most likely to be black male

4. May show no disability until stopping diazepam use

29. After chronic amphetamine use, abrupt withdrawal is likely to cause which of the following symptoms?

   1. Seizures
   2. Delirium
   3. Formication
   4. Sleep disturbance

30. In amphetamine delusional disorder, the patient is likely to show:

   1. Paranoid delusions
   2. Craving for food
   3. Tactile hallucinations
   4. Excessive REM sleep

31. During cocaine withdrawal, which of the following symptoms can be anticipated?

   1. Cardiac arrhythmias
   2. Desire for sleep, often with insomnia
   3. Delirium
   4. Depression

32. Which of the following statements about L-alpha-acetylmethadol are correct?

   1. Similar in action to methadone
   2. Dispensed only three times a week
   3. May cause nervousness and stimulation
   4. Withdrawal syndrome much shorter than methadone

33. Which of the following symptoms are characteristic of phencyclidine intoxication?

   1. Elevated blood pressure
   2. Pinpoint pupils
   3. Vertical nystagmus
   4. Hematuria

34. Which of the following statements about psychedelic drug use are correct?

   1. Tolerance quickly develops if used frequently
   2. Tolerance persists for extended period after drug use stopped
   3. No withdrawal phenomena when stopped after chronic use
   4. Cross-tolerance between LSD and amphetamines

35. Which of the following statements about LSD flashbacks are correct?

   1. Often triggered by marijuana use
   2. Usually cease within a few months of stopping hallucinogen
   3. Often pleasant to the hallucinogen user
   4. Subject may intentionally induce

36. When children of alcoholics are compared with controls in adopted-out studies, which of the following statements are correct?

    1. Six times higher incidence of psychopathology in children of alcoholics
    2. Three times risk of psychopathology in daughters of alcoholics
    3. Ten times higher risk of alcoholism in sons of alcoholics
    4. Four times rate of alcoholism in sons of alcoholics

37. Which of the following statements about alcohol metabolism are correct?

    1. In the liver, alcohol is metabolized to acetic acid
    2. When exposed to air, alcohol is broken down to acetic acid
    3. Disulfiram blocks the enzymatic breakdown to acetic acid
    4. A large proportion of alcohol ingested is expired in the breath

38. Which of the following statements about alcohol absorption are valid?

    1. Surgical removal of the pylorus allows more rapid absorption of alcohol
    2. Most alcohol is absorbed through the gastric mucosa
    3. Secretion of gastric mucus induced by high concentration of alcohol delays absorption
    4. The longer the alcohol remains in the blood, the greater the effect

39. Which of the following statements about the treatment of chronic alcoholics are correct?

    1. It is essential to face them with the physical consequences of their drinking during the first interview
    2. It is necessary to discuss frankly the patient's drinking patterns when initially interviewed
    3. Family history of alcoholism is irrelevant in the individual treatment prognosis
    4. The alcoholic's denial often makes the patient unavailable for treatment

40. Which of the following statements are applicable to alcohol idiosyncratic intoxication?

    1. Amnesia for time of intoxication
    2. Behavioral changes usually last several days
    3. Occurs within minutes of drinking
    4. Hallucinations occur in state of clear consciousness

41. Which of the following are likely to be shown by patients with alcoholic hallucinosis?

    1. Hallucinatory voices commenting unfavorably
    2. Underlying schizophrenic illness

3. Consciousness not impaired
4. No evidence of delusional thinking

42. Which of the following statements about alcoholics are correct?

    1. Suicidal behavior is common after personal loss
    2. High incidence of alcohol abuse in patients who commit suicide
    3. Alcohol tends to worsen depression
    4. Alcoholics who threaten suicide usually do not kill themselves

43. Which of the following would indicate alcohol dependence?

    1. Persistent drinking, even though worsens gastric ulcers
    2. Job efficiency impaired due to repeated hangovers
    3. Several unsuccessful attempts to cut down on drinking
    4. Family history of alcoholism

44. Chronic alcoholism is associated with:

    1. Retrobulbar optic neuropathy
    2. Caudate calcification
    3. Cerebellar anterior lobe degeneration
    4. Acoustic neuroma

45. Valid statements about the Wernicke-Korsakoff syndrome include:

    1. Direct toxic effect of alcohol on the neural system
    2. Short-term memory loss characteristic
    3. Thiamine produces reversal of dementia
    4. Associated with mammillary body necrosis

46. Which of the following statements about alcoholics withdrawing from alcohol are true?

    1. Overhydration more likely than dehydration
    2. Well-nourished patients should receive vitamins
    3. Often dependent also on other CNS depressants
    4. Withdrawal syndrome followed by insomnia

47. Alcoholics using disulfiram should avoid using:

    1. Aftershave
    2. Tricyclic antidepressants
    3. Cough syrup
    4. Pickled herring

48. Which of the following statements about disulfiram treatment of chronic alcoholism are correct?

    1. Indicated when the patient will not comply with other treatments
    2. Indicated in patients with Korsakoff syndrome
    3. Used where hepatic cirrhosis is present
    4. May be used in patients with antisocial personality disorder

49. Which of the following statements about the treatment of chronic alcoholism with disulfiram are correct?

    1. Alcohol dehydrogenase is inhibited
    2. Aldehyde accumulation causes vasodilation and hypotension
    3. Indicated in alcohol-induced dementia
    4. Treatment benefit is not dose-related

50. Which of the following statements about Alcoholics Anonymous are correct?

    1. Closely integrated with mental health services in most areas
    2. Control is primarily through group support
    3. Goal is a socially acceptable level of alcohol intake
    4. Typical attendance is several times per week

ANSWERS AND EXPLANATIONS

1. (3) A *physical withdrawal syndrome* occurs when a drug has become necessary to maintain homeostasis, usually after months of use and doses above therapeutic level. Abrupt stoppage of commonly used drugs such as narcotics, benzodiazepines, barbiturates, and alcohol can result in seizures, delirium, and cardiovascular collapse. (*CTP 1580. Har 423, 709. APA 818.*)

2. (3) In acute opioid overdose, the drug of choice is naloxone HCl (Narcan), 0.4–2.0 mg, preferably IV, every 2 to 3 minutes, to a maximum dose of 10 mg. Naloxone is an opioid antagonist that blocks opioid receptors. Other opioid antagonists are nalorphine and levellorphane. In an opioid withdrawal procedure, naltrexone HCl (Trexan), clonidine, and methadone may be used as they have longer acting effects. (*CTP 656-57. APA 336.*)

3. (2) Heroin addicts who are pregnant should be maintained on low-dose methadone (10–40 mg a day) to prevent withdrawal and uncontrolled use of narcotics and possible miscarriage and fetal death. (*CTP 684. APA 334.*)

4. (2) Heroin withdrawal symptoms are similar to a influenza-like syndrome along with anxiety and dysphoria. Physical symptoms include yawning, sweating, rhinorrhea, lacrimation, pupillary dilation, piloerection, hypertension, waves of gooseflesh, twitching movements, deep muscle and joint pains, nausea, diarrhea, vomiting, abdominal pains, fever, and hot and cold flashes. (*CTP 650. APA 331.*)

5. (1) The *pentobarbital challenge test*, 200 mg, is used to determine the starting dose of phenobarbital needed for barbiturate withdrawal and detoxification. If the patient falls asleep on 200 mg, no detoxification is required. If there are no signs of drug effect or intoxication, an extreme tolerance is present; therefore, 1,000–1,200 mg of phenobarbital initially over 24 hours may be needed, with a 10% reduction each day thereafter. If the 200 mg test dose produces slurred speech, ataxia, and intoxication, then a mild degree of tolerance is present; 400–600 mg of phenobarbital per day would be indicated to start withdrawal. If lateral nystagmus with no other signs of intoxication develop, then a marked degree of tolerance is present and 600–1000 mg per day would be the estimated requirement. (*CTP 668. APA 329. Har 424.*)

6. (2) Cocaine blocks neuronal dopamine, serotonin, and norepinephrine reuptake. With prolonged cocaine use and abuse, a delusional psychosis similar to paranoid schizophrenia may develop. (*CTP 668-73. APA 339.*)

7. (4) There are two groups of hallucinogens based on chemical structure:

    1. Indolealkylamines (resembles 5HT); includes LSD, DMT (methyltryptamine), psilocin, psilocybin.
    2. Phenylethylamines; includes mescaline (from peyote cactus), 2,5-dimethoxyamphetamine (DMA), 3,4-methylenedioxyamphetamine (MDA), and 3,4-methylenedioxymethamphetamine (MDMA).

    Symptoms of hallucinogenic drug use include dilated pupils, blurring of vision, sweating, incoordination, increased blood pressure, tachycardia, tremors, hyperreflexia, and mood changes ranging from euphoria to anxiety as well as visual illusions and perceptual changes (i.e., micropsia, synesthesias). Tolerance and cross-tolerance can develop. There are no withdrawal phenomena, and they are not reinforcers to other drugs. (*CTP 677. APA 344. Har 430-32.*)

8. (1) *Phencyclidine* ("angel dust," "crystal," "hog") *toxicity* induces organic mental disorders, intoxication, delirium, delusional mood, and flashback disorders with physical problems related to high blood pressure, muscle rigidity, ataxia, coma, nystagmus (particularly vertical), and dilated pupils. Treatment is with IV diazepam as the drug of first choice. Propranolol can be used for an adrenergic crisis, and haloperidol is effective for psychotic and disruptive behavior. Elimination of the drugs is enhanced by ammonium chloride in the acute stage and later by ascorbic acid. Environmental stimuli should be kept to a minimum. The urine is positive for PCP up to seven days, but there can be false negatives. (See question 33 for further information.) (*CTP 675-77. APA 343. Har 428.*)

9. (5) *Benzotropine* (Cogentin) has atropine-like side effects; dilated pupils, dry mouth, urinary retention, restlessness, confusion, and toxic psychosis. (*CTP 696. APA 802, 815, 834.*)

    1. *Phenelzine*, a MAOI, reacts with tyramine-containing substances causing a "cheese reaction," which consists of sweating, palpitations, headache, and increased blood pressure resulting in a possible intracerebral hemorrhage.
    2. *Disulfiram* (Antabuse), if taken with alcohol, causes flushing, throbbing, sweating, thirst, respiratory difficulty, nausea, vomiting, tachycardia, hypotension, vertigo, blurred vision, and confusion. (See question 47 for the mechanism of action.)
    3. Common side effects of propranolol, a beta adrenergic receptor blocker, include depression, hypotension, and bradycardia.

4. Alprazolam, a benzodiazepine, causes sedation, impairment of performance, and dependency.

10. (3) During alcohol induced blackouts, or "amnestic disorder," there are periods of retrograde amnesia (short-term memory deficits), even though state of consciousness may not appear to be abnormal. (*CTP 691. APA 323.*)

11. (3) Medical complications of *chronic alcoholism* are gastric bleeding, gastritis, achlorhydria, gastric ulcers, chronic pancreatitis, fatty liver, hepatitis, cirrhosis, cardiomyopathy, lowered immune response, hypoglycemia (may result in sudden death), and inhibited vitamins and amino acids absorption. In males, testicular atrophy, feminine pubic hair pattern, breast enlargement, and impotency may occur; female alcoholics may show decreased menstruation and infertility. Fetal alcohol syndrome (growth retardation before or after birth, small head circumference, flattening of facial features, CNS problems) is likely to be present in infants of female alcoholics. (Refer to question 44 for further complications of chronic alcoholism.) (*APA 318–19. CTP 693–94.*)

12. (1) *Alcohol withdrawal delirium* (delirium tremens, DT's) is characterized by confusion, disorientation, fluctuating or clouded consciousness, perceptual disturbances, delusions, vivid hallucinations, agitation, insomnia, mild fever, and marked autonomic arousal. Problems may appear suddenly or two to three days after cessation or reduction of heavy drinking, with a peak at the fourth or fifth day. Symptoms may last four to five weeks, but in the majority of patients, problems subside after three days. About one-third who develop alcohol withdrawal seizures ("rum fits") go into delirium tremens. The best treatment is to prevent withdrawal by the use of benzodiazepines and a high-calorie, high-carbohydrate diet with supplemental vitamins. (*APA 323–24. CTP 697, 203–4. Har 708–10.*)

13. (3) Alcohol withdrawal occurs when there is a relative drop in blood alcohol levels; therefore, it can develop while still drinking. The patients are likely to show a coarse, fast-frequency generalized tremor that is made worse by motor activity or stress and is easily observed when the hands or tongue are extended. Withdrawal is manifested by autonomic hyperactivity (increased BP, tachycardia, sweating), malaise, vomiting with anxiety, depression, irritability, cognitive changes, and possible seizures. (*CTP 203–4. APA 323–24. Har 709.*)

14. (2) The preferred medications for the management of alcohol withdrawal delirium are the benzodiazepines (chlordiazepoxide, diazepam, lorazepam, oxazepam). Multivitamins, particularly thiamine, B$_{12}$, and folic acid, should be used. Thiamine IV or IM should be given prior to glucose loading. If seizures develop, use magnesium sulfate. Clonidine, propranolol, chloral hydrate, benzodiazepines, or barbiturates can be used depending on the total clinical picture. (*CTP 1434. APA 323–25. Har 709.*)

15. (B) Tolerance occurs when the same dosage of drug has a reduced effect and increased amounts of the drug are needed to achieve the desired effect. Physical dependence, the need to take the drug to prevent withdrawal, tends to develop in parallel with tolerance. (*Har 427. CTP 648–49.*)

16. (C) Heroin abusers tend to start in late teens and early 20s (most common 18–25 years old), with the majority in the mid-30s. There is a 3:1 male to female ratio. Suicide in abusers is three times greater than in the general population. They also have a 20 times greater death rate, as well as higher rates of hepatitis B and HIV III viral infections. (*APA 330. CTP 654–56.*)

17. (A) Therapeutic communities for substance abusers have as their goals a complete change of lifestyle and abstinence from drugs. If the patient's stay is more than 90 days, there is a long-term decrease in illicit drug use, antisocial behavior, and arrests, and increased employment. With a 12-month stay, subjects fare even better at five years post-program follow-up. (*APA 336–37. CTP 661–63.*)

18. (C) Opioid addicts who are pregnant present special risks as high doses of narcotics (especially methadone) can lead to fetal problems on withdrawal or during delivery. (*CTP 684. APA 334.*)

19. (B) Withdrawal convulsions can occur with alcohol, certain benzodiazepines, and barbiturates. (Refer to questions 1, 12, and 20.) (*CTP 1579–82. APA 818. Har 709.*)

20. (E) Drugs that can cause seizures are phencyclidine, cocaine, alcohol, lithium, amphetamine, meperidine, and benzodiazepines. (*CTP 648, 668–77. Har 420, 425.*)

21. (A) Heavy marijuana users have an "amotivational syndrome," characterized by passivity, decreased drive, diminished goal-directed activity, decreased memory, fatigue, apathy, and poor problem solving. Physiological changes consist of an increased heart rate, blood pressure (therefore problems with those who have cardiovascular diseases), and chronic obstructive lung disorders. Cannabinoids can be detected in urine up to 21 days after stopping in chronic users, due to redistribution in fat, but are usually detected from one to five days in occasional users. (*CTP 673–74. APA 347–49. Har 426.*)

22. (E) U.S. enlisted soldiers addicted to opioids in RVN did not follow the pattern of addicted civilians: on return to U.S.; the great majority no longer used the drug (heroin). (*CTP 652–54.*)

23. **(C)** Opioid toxicity or overdose should be suspected in any undiagnosed coma patient or patients with respiratory depression (pulmonary edema), shock (hypothermia), pupillary construction, and needle marks. Grand mal seizures can occur with meperidine overdose. (*CTP 650–57. APA 331.*)

24. **(E)** Medications used in the rehabilitation (maintenance) of opioid-dependent patients are methadone (as a substitute for opiates), a combination of naltraxone and clonidine (long-acting antagonists) and L-alpha-acetylmethadol (LAAM, an agonist similar to methadone but longer half-life). (See question number 2 for overdose information.) (*CTP 659–61. APA 330–36.*)

25. **(A)** Sedative, hypnotic, or anxiolytic drugs have a high index of therapeutic safety but can be abused, especially in combination with other substances such as alcohol. Duration of drug use (use is usually for short-term adjustments), the amount of drug use, and the role of elimination of drug and metabolites, all are factors in producing tolerance or dependency. (*CTP 664–68. APA 328–29. Har 424–25.*)

26. **(E)** Barbiturate withdrawal (especially short acting) usually results in weakness, insomnia, anxiety, tremulousness, abdominal discomfort, nausea and vomiting. With preexisting cardiovascular problems, there may be fatal reactions. Seizures generally precede delirium. Symptoms are most marked with secobarbital and least with phenobarbital withdrawal (due to its long half-life). (*CTP 666–67. APA 328–30. Har 423–24.*)

27. **(E)** (*CTP 666–67. APA 328–30. Har 423–24.*)

28. **(C)** Diazepam has a high potential for abuse and dependence, which may develop over months (high doses) to years (low doses). Alcohol, opiates, or cocaine intake may precipitate overdose. The patient, if tolerant or dependent, may show no disability until several days later after stopping the use of diazepam when withdrawal symptoms develop. (*APA 328–30. CTP 664–68. Har 425.*)

29. **(D)** Amphetamines or "speed" are stimulants with reinforcing effects similar to cocaine. Chronic amphetamine use causes tachycardia, elevated BP, pupillary dilation, agitation, elations, and hypervigilance. Adverse side effects include insomnia, fever, headaches, confusion, irritability, hostility, and visual hallucinations. (*CTP 671–72. APA 342–43. Har 423.*)

30. **(B)** Amphetamine and cocaine delusional disorders are very similar and can resemble paranoid schizophrenia. Common symptoms are paranoid delusions with distortions of body image and misperception of face, a predominance of visual and tactile hallucinations, confusion, incoherence, hyperactivity, and hypersexuality. (*CTP 669–70. APA 343. Har 419.*)

31. **(C)** Cocaine withdrawal has no specific physiological signs, but there are physical problems ("crash") that peak in two to four days. Depression and irritability can persist for weeks. These patients show a desire for sleep, often with insomnia, with disturbed sleep and increased dreaming, general fatigue, and suicidal ideation. Drug-seeking behavior usually occurs after being drug-free for a few days. (*CTP 671–72. APA 338. Har 421.*)

32. **(A)** Levo-alpha-acetylmethadol (LAAM) is an opioid agonist similar to methadone in action but with a longer half-life. Since it provides a longer time of suppression of withdrawal for 72–96 hours, it can be dispensed (30–80 mg) only three times per week and has less abuse potential due to its slow induction. LAAM may cause nervousness, overstimulation, and mood side effects. (*CTP 661. APA 334.*)

33. **(B)** Phencyclidine (PCP, "angel dust," developed in the 1950s for veterinary use) and related arycyclohexylamines have CNS stimulation, CNS depressant, hallucinogenic, and analgesic actions. Structurally related compounds are dexoxadrol, ketamine (Ketalar), and N-(1-[z-thienyl] cyclohexyl)-piperidine (TCP). PCP can be detected in the urine for several days after use. Prominent features of PCP use are increased blood pressure, heart rate, and vertical or horizontal nystagmus. There is decreased response to pain, ataxia, dysarthria, muscle rigidity, seizures, and hyperacusis. Individuals can have a serious catatonic syndrome, toxic psychosis, acute mental syndrome, or coma. Suicide is a risk. (See question number 8.) (*CTP 675–77. APA 343. Har 428.*)

34. **(B)** Repeated psychedelic drug use over an extended period of time can quickly result in tolerance. There is a cross-tolerance with LSD, mescaline, and psilocybin, but not between LSD and amphetamines or delta9-THC. There is no known withdrawal pattern. (See question 7 for further information.) (*CTP 677–79. APA 343–45. Har 430–32.*)

35. **(E)** LSD flashbacks are common, with 25% of users experiencing an episode and with 5% there will be a severe reaction. Flashbacks usually cease in a few months after stopping the drug use. The most common type of flashbacks are hallucinations of formed objects (face, geometric), sounds, voices, flashes of color, false perceptions of movement, positive afterimages, and trails of images from moving objects. Most of the flashback symptoms are enjoyable. It is rare for the drugs to produce any lethal effects. Chromosomal damage from the use of hallucinogens or from marijuana use is still questionable. (*CTP 678. APA 344. Har 431.*)

36. **(D)** There is a strong genetic factor seen in alcoholics and their families. Sons of male alcoholics are more vulnerable than daughters and become alcoholic four times

more often than children of nonalcoholics, even when they are not raised by their biological parents. Monozygotic twins have twice the concordance rate for alcoholism as compared with dizygotic twins of the same sex. Further, family alcoholism results in earlier onset, more antisocial features, worse medical problems, and a poorer prognosis. (*CTP 696. APA 320. Har 703.*)

37. (A) Alcohol metabolism and excretion begin immediately after absorption. Kidneys and lungs excrete about one-tenth of the alcohol ingested unchanged, whereas the rest undergoes a fairly constant rate of oxidation. The liver is the main site for alcohol catabolism. Disulfiram inhibits the enzyme aldehyde dehydrogenase and alcohol ingestion causes a toxic reaction due to the acetaldehyde accumulation in the blood. (*CTP 687–88.*)

38. (B) Alcohol absorption is slowed by food, but increased by water, especially if carbonated. Alcohol goes directly into the bloodstream from the stomach and it is distributed throughout all tissues of the body. If stomach alcohol concentration becomes too high, mucus is secreted and the pyloric valve closes, thereby slowing absorption. (*CTP 688.*)

39. (C) Treatment of chronic alcoholics is the treatment of a chronic relapsing illness. A nonjudgmental approach needs to be used toward slips, drinking patterns, and the patient's denial. Education and treatment of the family are essential. Emphasis on support groups, self-help aspects of treatment, especially AA's 12-step program, aids resocialization and acceptance of an identity as a recovering person.

    Treatment of underlying psychiatric disorders is important. About two-thirds of chronic alcoholics have additional psychiatric problems such as depression, anxiety disorder, and attention deficit. Those alcoholic patients with a primary or secondary psychiatric illness have an increased suicide rate compared with those who do not have any additional psychiatric diagnosis. (*APA 325–28. Har 705–8.*)

40. (B) Alcohol idiosyncratic intoxication, also known as "pathological intoxication," is manifested by the sudden onset of marked behavior changes after consumption of a small amount of alcohol: these symptoms usually last for a few hours, terminate in prolonged sleep, and the individual is unable to recall the episode. There can be blind, unfocused, assaultive behavior, as well as suicidal ideation and attempts. (*CTP 1434. APA 323.*)

41. (B) Alcohol hallucinosis is a rare withdrawal symptom in which the patient experiences vivid visual or auditory voices commenting unfavorably. It usually lasts 48 hours, but may go on for one week or more. The symptoms occur shortly after cessation (within a day or two) or after the reduction of heavy ingestion of alcohol. Pa-

tients are likely to show fear, anxiety, and agitation. The hallucinations are not part of the alcohol withdrawal delirium, and the sensorium is clear. (*APA 324. CTP 695. Har 381.*)

42. (A) Alcoholism is the third largest health problem after heart disease and cancer. In males 25–44 years old, alcohol plays a major role in all four leading causes of death: accidents, homicides, suicides, and alcoholic cirrhosis. The chronic use of alcohol produces psychological, interpersonal, and medical problems, which include violence, absence from work, loss of job, and legal difficulties. Alcohol is a factor associated with at least 50% of traffic fatalities, 50% of homicides, and 25% of suicides. (*CTP 695. Har 701.*)

43. (A) Alcohol dependence is characterized by the inability to cut down and stop drinking, despite repeated efforts to control drinking ("going on the wagon"), binges, and amnesia periods, and continued drinking while knowing a serious physical condition is being exacerbated by alcohol. (See question 42.) (*CTP 686–87. Har 701.*)

44. (B) *Chronic alcoholism* is associated with retrobulbar optic neuropathy, cerebellar anterior lobe degeneration, encephalopathy (Wernicke's), subdural hematoma, amnestic disorder (Korsakoff's syndrome), dementia, peripheral neuropathy, pancreatitis, esophageal varices, duodenal ulcer, cardiomyopathy, pulmonary infections (especially tuberculosis), cirrhosis, and fetal alcohol syndrome. (*CTP 693. Har 710.*)

45. (C) *Wernicke-Korsakoff syndrome* manifests by an abrupt-onset encephalopathy, with truncal ataxia, ophthalmoplegia (particularly 6th cranial nerve), nystagmus, and mental confusion. It is believed to be due to thiamine deficiency (malabsorption syndrome) and may lead to death, psychosis, chronic amnestic disorder, and severe anterograde amnesia (memory not transferred from short- to long-term memory). Pathological examination reveals necrosis in the brainstem, diencephalon, and mammillary bodies. (*CTP 639. APA 323. Har 363.*)

46. (E) Physical symptoms of withdrawal from alcohol usually occur 6–48 hours after last drink, subside in 5–7 days without treatment, but irritability and insomnia may last 10 days or longer. Nutritional and vitamin deficiencies are common even if the individual appears well nourished. The patient must be watched for overhydration especially during IV fluid replacement. (See question 13 for further details.) (*APA 323–24. CTP 1434. Har 709.*)

47. (B) Disulfiram (Antabuse) results in a severe reaction if alcohol is ingested; therefore, one must avoid using any products containing alcohol such as aftershave lotions, cough syrups, sauces, and vinegar. Disulfiram com-

pletely inhibits the enzyme aldehyde dehydrogenase, causing a toxic reaction due to acetaldehyde accumulation in the blood. (*CTP 687. Har 707.*)

48. **(D)** Disulfiram treatment is an important adjunct to the rehabilitation program with the alcoholic. The patient only has to make the decision about not drinking, and it gives the individual time to think about the impulse to drink. Therefore, the patient must be healthy (due to the side effects with alcohol), highly motivated, and cooperative. (*APA 326. CTP 698. Har 707.*)

49. **(C)** Disulfiram is taken in a 250–500 mg dose per day. Higher doses can be toxic, resulting in psychosis, memory impairment, and confusion without offering any better control. (See questions 47–48.) (*CTP 687. APA 325–26.*)

50. **(C)** Alcoholics Anonymous (AA) is a voluntary, supportive fellowship, self-help group, and is worldwide. It was founded in 1936 by Bill Wilson. Meetings provide acceptance, understanding, forgiveness, confrontation, and a means of positive identification. Programs consist of 12 steps and the use of sponsors. AA is not tied to any religion, but does allow for spiritual reevaluation. (See question 39.) (*APA 327. CTP 1529. Har 701, 707.*)

3

ADULT PSYCHIATRY
Anxiety Disorders, Schizophrenia, Mood Disorders, and Personality Disorders

DIRECTIONS: Select the best single response for questions 1 through 21.

1. The most effective management of a patient with somatization disorder would be:

    1. Long-term care by the primary physician
    2. Referral for psychoanalysis
    3. Periodic crisis-focused psychotherapy
    4. Regular use of safe placebo as symptoms occur
    5. Sodium amytal interview

2. All of the following statements about patients with somatization disorder are correct except:

    1. Usually female
    2. Increased prevalence of antisocial personality disorder in first-degree male relatives
    3. Increased prevalence of somatization disorder in first-degree female relatives
    4. Patients are rarely disabled by the symptoms
    5. Similar symptoms in many medical disorders

3. All of the following statements about patients with panic disorders are correct except:

    1. Often go on to develop agoraphobia
    2. Attacks precipitated by low-dose yohimbine
    3. Monoamine oxidase inhibitors often block attacks
    4. Imipramine contraindicated with mitral valve prolapse
    5. Associated with temporal lobe epilepsy

4. Behavioral treatment of social phobia may include all of the following except:

    1. Social skills training
    2. In vivo exposure
    3. Gradual exposure *in imagination*
    4. Gentle supportive interpretation
    5. Implosion therapy

5. When bipolar disorder is designated type II, this indicates:

    1. Major depressive and manic episodes
    2. Major depressive and hypomanic episodes
    3. Dysthymic disorder and manic episodes
    4. Major depression superimposed on dysthymic disorder
    5. Major depression with melancholia

6. The following statements about patients with double depression are valid except:

    1. Less likely to have full recovery than patients with uncomplicated depression
    2. Relapse more likely than major depression
    3. May be present in one quarter of patients with disabling depression
    4. Poorer response to electroconvulsive therapy than uncomplicated depression
    5. Not caused by toxic or organic factors

7. All of the following statements about mania are correct except:

    1. Most frequent type of onset of bipolar disorder
    2. Speech may be incoherent
    3. Often angry, resentful, and hostile
    4. Cognitive organization maintained
    5. Frequent regressed behavior

8. In mild disorders, the following statements about cycling are correct except:

    1. Cycles tend to be longer in unipolar depression
    2. Cycles tend to get longer as disorder persists
    3. Rapid cyclers are less responsive to lithium
    4. Rapid cyclers are more often female
    5. Sexes are equal in cycle duration

9. Which disability is least associated with high suicide risk?

    1. Terminal cancer
    2. Schizophrenia

3. Major depression
4. Substance abuse
5. Personality disorder

10. Which diagnostic groups have the highest rate of suicide?

   1. Depression-schizophrenia
   2. Organic brain disorder–depression
   3. Terminal medical illness–depression
   4. Depression-alcoholism
   5. Personality disorder–depression

11. In response to your question, a school teacher states that the meaning of "people who live in glass houses should not throw stones" is "you might break the glass." This response is an example of:

   1. Autistic thinking
   2. Concrete thinking
   3. Poverty of thought
   4. Poverty of content
   5. Tangentiality

12. Negative symptoms in schizophrenia could include all of the following except:

   1. Flat affect
   2. Apathy
   3. Poverty of thought
   4. Nihilistic delusions
   5. Anhedonia

13. Computed tomography studies have shown which of the following abnormal findings most often in schizophrenia?

   1. Pineal calcification
   2. Caudate-putamen atrophy
   3. Aqueductal dilatation
   4. Lateral ventricle enlargement
   5. Increased frontal density

14. Hypnogogic hallucinations are:

   1. False perception of insects crawling on the skin
   2. False perceptions when falling asleep
   3. A sensation that is perceived in a different sensory modality
   4. False perceptions associated with alcohol abuse
   5. Misperceptions with real external stimuli

15. A psychotic syndrome similar to paranoid schizophrenia is likely to be induced by:

   1. Dantrolene
   2. Phenytoin
   3. Amphetamines
   4. Alprazolam
   5. Salicylates

16. All of the following are characteristics of a paranoid personality disorder except:

   1. Fixed systematic delusions
   2. Oversensitivity to fantasied slights
   3. Social isolation
   4. Reluctance to seek treatment
   5. Rejection by others

17. All of the following statements apply to patients with factitious disorder except:

   1. Deliberate mimicking of illness
   2. Goal to become medical patient
   3. Tend to have multiple visitors
   4. Resist referral for psychiatric care
   5. Frequently leave against medical advice

18. As a group, patients with personality disorders show all of the following except:

   1. Symptoms usually recognizable before adulthood
   2. Repetitious, maladaptive ways of coping
   3. Behavior distressing to others
   4. Behavior that is ego-dystonic
   5. Tendency to blame others

19. All of the following statements apply to the person with a schizoid personality disorder except:

   1. Does not enjoy close relationships
   2. Hypersensitive to criticism
   3. Preoccupied with inner world psychologically
   4. Chooses solitary activities
   5. No cognitive distortion

20. Which feature most clearly differentiates narcissistic from borderline personality disorder?

   1. Splitting used as a defense mechanism
   2. Lacking in empathy for others
   3. Feelings of inner emptiness
   4. Reacts with unreasonable rage
   5. Prone to show psychotic decompensation

21. The defense mechanism most characteristic of patients with borderline personality disorder is:

   1. Undoing
   2. Denial
   3. Splitting
   4. Displacement
   5. Dissociation

DIRECTIONS: For questions 22 through 80, one or more of the alternatives given are correct. After you decide which alternatives are correct, record your answer according to the following key.

(A) if alternatives 1, 2 and 3 only are correct.
(B) if alternatives 1 and 3 only are correct.

(C) if alternatives 2 and 4 only are correct.
(D) if alternative 4 only is correct.
(E) if all four alternatives are correct

22. In the management of panic attacks, which of the following statements apply?

    1. Imipramine produces blockage of panic attacks after four to five weeks of treatment
    2. Antidepressant dosages required for effective treatment are higher than with depression
    3. Patients tend to be sensitive to the stimulant effect of antidepressants
    4. Anticipatory anxiety responds quickly to antidepressant medication

23. Panic attacks may be induced by:

    1. Cocaine intoxication
    2. Marijuana abuse
    3. Alcohol withdrawal
    4. Hyperthyroidism

24. Epidemiological studies regarding panic disorders show which of the following?

    1. Over 15% first-degree relatives have panic attacks
    2. Agoraphobia twice as common in females
    3. Onset usually age 15 to 25
    4. Patients do not have sleep disruption due to panic attacks

25. Which of the following are consistent with a diagnosis of conversion disorder?

    1. Coexistent similar organically caused illness
    2. Muscle contraction and atrophy
    3. Marked secondary gain
    4. Symptom onset following stress

26. Factors predisposing to conversion disorder include:

    1. Family incidence of conversion disorder
    2. Serious medical illness
    3. Dependent personality disorder
    4. Young adult

27. In considering seizures as a manifestation of conversion disorder, which of the following statements apply?

    1. Not diagnosed when patient has proven epilepsy
    2. Marked secondary gain supports conversion disorder diagnosis
    3. La belle indifference indicates conversion disorder
    4. Conversion disorder patients rarely hurt themselves during a hysterical seizure

28. In patients with multiple personalities:

    1. Frequently there is a history of physical and sexual abuse in childhood

    2. On mental status examination, patient may show no abnormalities other than amnesia for periods of time
    3. Illness tends to be chronic, lifelong
    4. Onset is usually between ages 20 and 30

29. Clinical manifestations of psychogenic fugue include:

    1. Loss of memory with distress over this loss
    2. Abrupt onset of symptoms
    3. Fugue patients appear odd or strange to people around them
    4. Patients assume new identity

30. In differentiating psychogenic amnesia from organic amnesia, which of the following are correct?

    1. Deficit in recent memory in both
    2. Amnesia for personal identity is usually psychogenic
    3. Psychogenic amnesia clears gradually
    4. Amytal interview worsens organic amnesia symptoms

31. Characteristics of the premenstrual syndrome include:

    1. Symptoms become less severe in older women
    2. Higher incidence of suicide around menses
    3. Dysmenorrhea commoner in older women
    4. Diagnosed when confirmed by two prospective cycle ratings

32. Fear of impending death, sweating, trembling, and change in respiratory rate may be symptoms of which of the following?

    1. Cocaine withdrawal
    2. Generalized anxiety disorder
    3. Hypoglycemia
    4. Myocardial infarction

33. Disabling fears of leaving home may be a manifestation of:

    1. Paranoid schizophrenia
    2. Post-traumatic stress disorder
    3. Major depression
    4. Agoraphobia

34. Which of the following treatments may be used effectively in obsessive compulsive disorder?

    1. Clomipramine
    2. Leukotomy
    3. Exposure in vivo plus response prevention
    4. Desipramine

35. Which of the following statements about obsessive compulsive disorder are correct?

    1. Higher incidence in relatives of Tourette's disorder patients
    2. Twice as common in men
    3. Anal sadistic phase disturbance
    4. Better prognosis with early age of onset

36. Which of the following statements about patients with post-traumatic stress disorder are valid?

    1. Stress due to aging may activate the syndrome
    2. Full syndrome usually starts immediately after the stress
    3. Group therapy often more effective than individual therapy
    4. Alprazolam often beneficial

37. Which of the following symptoms could be manifestations of generalized anxiety disorder?

    1. Difficulty maintaining concentration
    2. Problems falling asleep
    3. Loss of train of thought
    4. Tachycardia

38. Which of the following sleep stage abnormalities are seen in patients with major depression?

    1. Decreased stage 4 sleep
    2. Shortened initial non-REM period
    3. Increased REM density
    4. REM sleep rebound after deprivation

39. Characteristics of melancholia include:

    1. Marked psychomotor agitation
    2. Depression more severe in the evening
    3. Early wakening
    4. Poor response to antidepressant medication

40. All of the following statements about postpartum blues are correct except:

    1. Most prominent two to three weeks postpartum
    2. Most severe in multigravid women
    3. Usually clears spontaneously
    4. Increasing severity with further pregnancies

41. Organic disorders that may present as a depressive disorder include:

    1. Myxedma
    2. Early dementia
    3. Pancreatic carcinoma
    4. Wernicke's encephalophathy

42. Medications that commonly produce depression include:

    1. Propranolol
    2. Estrogen
    3. Guanethidine
    4. Aminophylline

43. A false positive dexamethasone test may occur in which of the following?

    1. Anorexia nervosa
    2. Phenytoin use
    3. Acute withdrawal from alcohol
    4. Pregnancy

44. In patients with seasonal affective disorder, which of the following apply?

    1. Winter depression is likely to be followed by summer hypomania
    2. Respond well to antidepressant medication
    3. Typically increased eating and sleep during depressive phase
    4. Dexamethasone suppression test usually positive during depression

45. Which of the following statements apply to the concept of learned helplessness?

    1. Based on Harlow's primate research
    2. Disturbance of cognitive processing leads to depression
    3. Reflects fixation at the oral stage
    4. Outcomes are independent of responses

46. According to Arnold Beck, which of the following apply to depression?

    1. Depression results from distortions of cognition
    2. Depression-prone people tend to see the world negatively
    3. Depression-prone people view themselves as being defective
    4. Depression-prone people have learned helplessness

47. Which of the following statements about affective disorders are correct?

    1. In male-female lifetime prevalence rates, greater discrepancy in bipolar disorder
    2. Peak incidence of onset of unipolar disorder is age 45 to 55
    3. Peak incidence of onset of schizoaffective disorder is age 30 to 40
    4. With late onset bipolar disorder, manic episodes are more likely to be mild

48. Disorders more common in women include:

    1. Somatization disorder
    2. Simple phobia
    3. Unipolar depression
    4. Antisocial personality

49. When patients with major depression and bipolar disorder depression are compared, which of the following statements are correct?

    1. Bipolar disorder depression is more common in females by the ratio of two to one
    2. Later peak age of onset in major depression

3. Family history of major depression twice as common in major depression patients compared with bipolar depressed
4. No relationship is present between race and bipolar disorder or major depression

50. Which of the following statements about patients with major depression are correct?

1. Peak age of onset in 20s
2. Male-female ratio about equal
3. Twice as common in black population
4. Lifetime prevalence five to ten times bipolar

51. Mania may be caused by:

1. L-dopa
2. Amphetamines
3. Isoniazid
4. Encephalitis

52. In managing an exhausted, confused manic patient, appropriate emergency treatment would be:

1. Electroconvulsive therapy
2. Lithium carbonate
3. Haloperidol
4. Carbamazepine

53. In patients who have unipolar depression, showing marked somatic and nihilistic delusions, the appropriate management could include:

1. Haloperidol
2. Electroconvulsive therapy
3. Tricyclic antidepressant
4. Lithium carbonate

54. Which of the following groups have a higher rate of suicide?

1. Males as compared with females
2. Elderly as compared with adolescents
3. Unmarried as compared with married
4. Female physicians as compared with general population

55. Which of the following statements about the incidence of suicide in the United States are correct?

1. Suicide rates in females have steadily increased from 1965 to the present
2. Suicide is the third leading cause of death over age 65
3. Black females have higher suicide rates than white females
4. Divorced people have higher suicide rates than unmarried

56. Which of the following factors indicate increased suicide risk?

1. Previous suicide attempts
2. Telling others of suicide intent
3. Substance abuse
4. Family history of suicide

57. Which of the following circumstances would suggest a higher risk in a patient who has made a suicide attempt?

1. More than one means used to carry out the suicide
2. Suicide attempt within the sight of a family member
3. Suicide note left
4. Open expression of anger toward family

58. In the management of an acutely suicidal patient, which of the following would be appropriate?

1. Electroconvulsive therapy
2. Constant observation
3. Antidepressant medication
4. Consent of spouse for involuntary hospitalization

59. Which of the following statements apply to patients with hysteroid dysphoria?

1. Sensitivity to rejection
2. More responsive to tricyclic antidepressants
3. Fatigue and hypersomnia
4. Poor appetite with weight loss

60. Eugen Bleuler is noted for which of the following clinical advances?

1. Distinguishing manic depressive illness from the psychoses
2. Defining schizophrenia as a group of thought disorders
3. First pointing out the early age of onset of schizophrenia
4. Indicating that not all patients with schizophrenia have a deteriorating course

61. The hypothesis that excess dopaminergic activity is related to the development of schizophrenia is supported by:

1. Similarity of bromocriptine-induced psychosis to schizophrenia
2. Similarity of amphetamine-induced psychosis to paranoid schizophrenia
3. Similarity between antipsychotic potency and neuroleptic affinity for dopamine receptors
4. Antipsychotic effect of reserpine

62. Genetic studies have shown the risk of schizophrenia to be:

1. 60–80% where both parents are schizophrenic
2. 10% in first-degree relatives of schizophrenics
3. 85–100% where monozygotic twin is schizophrenic
4. 1% of general population

63. Which of the following statements about schizophrenia are correct?

    1. Highest incidence in lower socioeconomic groups
    2. Diagnosed twice as often in females
    3. Onset in males tends to be earlier than in females
    4. More frequent in industrialized society

64. When paranoid schizophrenia is compared with other schizophrenia subtypes, which of the following statements are valid?

    1. Tends to start at an older age
    2. More obvious social regression
    3. Less thinking disorganization
    4. Higher incidence in males

65. Valid statements about delusional (paranoid) disorder include:

    1. Systematized nonbizarre delusions
    2. Not considered a psychotic disorder
    3. Later onset than schizophrenia
    4. Prominent auditory hallucinations

66. Stupor, mutism, rigidity, and negativism are symptoms that may be caused by:

    1. Major depression
    2. Schizophrenia
    3. Phencyclidine toxicity
    4. Neuroleptic overdose

67. Which of the following statements apply to schizoaffective disorder?

    1. Symptoms do not respond to lithium
    2. Prognosis better than schizophrenia
    3. Good response to antidepressants
    4. Earlier onset than unipolar depression

68. In working with schizophrenics and their families, which of the following statements are correct?

    1. Family therapy is more effective in preventing relapse than is medication
    2. Families should be supportive, but not overinvolved
    3. That patients' severity of psychotic symptoms predicts the likelihood of relapse
    4. Psychosocial treatment should be long term

69. Which of the following would suggest a good prognosis in a schizophrenic patient?

    1. Patient has a job
    2. Patient is depressed
    3. Patient is married
    4. Onset in adolescence

70. The patient with intermittent explosive disorder is likely to show which of the following?

    1. Repeated episodic loss of control
    2. Normal behavior between episodes
    3. Past arrests for traffic violations
    4. Lack of guilt or remorse for behavior

71. Antisocial personality disorder in males has a higher incidence under which of the following circumstances?

    1. Father is an alcoholic
    2. Mother has somatization disorder
    3. Mother was neglectful and indifferent
    4. Childhood attention deficit disorder

72. Which of the following statements about patients with antisocial personality disorder are correct?

    1. Self-help groups are more effective than individual psychotherapy
    2. Increased incidence of suicidal behavior
    3. Symptoms present in early adolescence
    4. Greater incidence of parental loss during childhood compared with other personality disorders

73. Characteristics of pathological gamblers include:

    1. Alcoholism more common in parents
    2. Typically unmarried and socially isolated
    3. Compulsive gambling began in adolescence
    4. Equal sex incidence

74. Characteristics of people with self-defeating personality disorder include:

    1. Provoke anger and rejection
    2. Reluctant to enter treatment
    3. Often involved in abusive relationship
    4. Frequently depressed and hopeless

75. Which of the following statements apply to malingering?

    1. Change of physical function due to emotional disorder
    2. Obsessive preoccupation with physical features
    3. Patient seeks medical investigation or hospitalization
    4. Patient seeks some recognizable benefits

76. Manifestations of Type A personality include:

    1. More successful than Type B persons
    2. Constantly trying to achieve
    3. Coronary heart disease higher in outwardly hostile
    4. Can be diagnosed by speech patterns

77. Which of the following statements would apply to the patient with a passive aggressive personality?

    1. Forgets responsibilities
    2. Depressed and hopeless
    3. Discontented, irritable, resistant
    4. Often involved in abusive relationship

78. Which of the following statements about borderline personality disorder are correct?

1. Increased prevalence of schizophrenia in first-degree relatives
2. Depressive symptoms are short-lived and rarely last more than a day
3. Socially are "loners"
4. Respond to frustration with overwhelming rage

79. In the psychotherapeutic treatment of the borderline patient, which of the following are likely to be problems?

1. Therapist countertransference
2. Regression by the patient
3. Splitting of the treatment team
4. Premature termination

80. Which of the following statements about patients with a borderline personality disorder are correct?

1. Does not desire friendships
2. Incapable of relating ambivalently
3. Does not respond well to neuroleptics
4. Frequent fear of abandonment

ANSWERS AND EXPLANATIONS

1. **(1)** Patients with a *somatization disorder* (Briquet's syndrome) give a history of many physical complaints (in the female often sexual dysfunctions) or believe that they are sickly. Complaints and problems begin before age 30 and persist for several years. Any medical care should be unified through one general medical physician who can provide consistent ongoing long-term supportive care, which may help avoid unnecessary surgery and medical procedures. (*CTP 1009-13. APA 544-46. Har 256-57.*)

2. **(4)** A somatization disorder is common in females (0.2–2%) but is less common in males. There is an increased prevalence (20%) of the disorder in the patient's first-degree relatives, with an increased family rate of marital problems, poor work performance, teenage delinquencies, alcohol problems, and sociopathy. There is also a high incidence of concurrent psychiatric disorders in patients. (*CTP 1009-13. APA 544-46. Har 256-57.*)

3. **(4)** In individuals with panic attacks, panic can be induced by sodium lactate infusion, 5% carbon dioxide in room air, or yohimbine. Similar symptoms of panic have been reported in temporal lobe epilepsy. There is a high incidence within families of individuals developing agoraphobia and mitral valve prolapse. In addition, relatives have similar positive and negative responses to certain tricyclic and MAOI treatment. (*APA 443-58. CTP 952-72. Har 235-41.*)

4. **(4)** The treatment of a patient with a social phobia consists of systematic desensitization, cognitive restructuring, and social skills training. (*APA 468. CTP 982-83. Har 238-39.*)

   Flooding (*implosion*) is a type of behavior therapy used in treating patients with phobias and other maladaptive anxiety. A stimulus that causes problems is presented in an intense form, either through imagination or in real life and is continued until the stimulus no longer produces the disabling anxiety.

5. **(2)** The major subtypes of bipolar disorders are depressed, manic, and mixed. Bipolar disorders can be divided into two types:

   Type I or Bipolar I is synonymous with the DSM-III-R criteria for bipolar disorder (manic depressive). There is a history of recurrent mania and hypomania, and distinct periods of major depressions. Overall, the patients reveal alternating episodes of elevated, expansive, or irritable moods accompanied by increased activity, pressure of speech, flight of ideas, grandiosity, decreased need for sleep, and/or distractibility. Usually, thinking process remains coherent but it may be tangential.

   Type II or Bipolar II refers to patients with major depressions and an absence of, or only mild, hypomanic episodes.

   Sixty to eighty percent of bipolar patients begin with mania episodes. The rate for bipolar is equal for males and females, starting at age 20 to early 30s. The lifetime prevalence is 1%. Sixty to seventy percent of the patients give a positive familial history of major depression. (*APA 406, 1025. Har 317. DSM-III-R 214. CTP 892-93.*)

6. **(4)** Double depression is present in patients who have a major depressive episode superimposed on an underlying chronic depression. This situation occurs in one-fourth of moderately to severely depressed patients. Recovery is only one-half as likely as compared with other depressions and relapses are two times more common for those who do not recover completely from both depressions. (*APA 408. CTP 1676. Har 1676.*)

7. **(4)** Manic episodes occur less frequently than depressions and represent a spectrum of euphoric and elated states with impaired social and familial behavior. "Delirious mania" is manifested by markedly hostile, aggressive, and destructive behavior. Some manic patients are also psychotic. (See question number 5 for additional information.) (*APA 412-14. CTP 904. Har 314-15.*)

8. **(2)** Rapid cycling occurs in patients when both mania and major depression episodes alternate rapidly from hour to hour, day to day, or week to week, and present with at least three or four episodes per year. Rapid cycling may be a complication of chronic antidepressant treatment. Recovery for patients with a mixed cyclic pattern takes one and one-half times longer than for those with pure depression and three times longer than for those with pure mania. Treatment for rapid cycling is nonspecific, but a trial of levothyroxine sodium (T_4), or carbamazepine can be used to supplement the effects of lithium. A new drug, not available in the U.S., clorgyline, a MAO-A inhibitor, may be effective. (*CTP 893-94, 1659-60. APA 413.*)

9. **(1)** The highest suicide risks are in males, adolescents, and the elderly, with those who are single, divorced, live alone, and with substance abuse (especially alcohol), major depression, schizophrenia, and impulsive character disorders. The lowest risk is with females, and those who are married, in their midyears, living in a rural area, and church goers. (*APA 1023-26. Har 744-45.*)

10. **(4)** Suicide is the ninth leading cause of death in U.S., making up 2% of all deaths annually. The highest rate of suicide is in old age, in individuals older than 65

years. Within the adolescent group, ages 15–24, suicide is the third leading cause of death. Two disorders associated with more than two-thirds of all suicides are affective illness (40–80%) and alcoholism (15–30%). There is an increased incidence of suicide in patients with schizophrenia, organic mental disorder, and other mental illnesses. (*APA 1024-26.*)

11. (2) *Concrete thinking* is literal, one dimensional, based on immediate experience rather than on abstraction or use of metaphors. (*APA 364-65. CTP 472, 561. Har 36.*)

Autistic thinking is distorted, self-centered, fantastic, and with no regard for reality.

Poverty of thought refers to limited responses and thinking.

Tangentiality is manifested by responses that are oblique or irrelevant to a question.

Circumstantiality is an indirect and delayed answer to a question.

Derailment is the loss of goal in thinking.

12. (4) Negative or passive symptoms in schizophrenia refer to the decrease in expression that affects the cognitive, emotional, and behavioral spheres of the individual. They consist of flat, blunted, or restricted affect; apathy; lack of feeling, emotion, interest, or concern; nihilistic delusion (nonexistence of the self, part of the self, or of some object in external reality); and anhedonia, the inability to experience pleasure (as contrasted to hedonism). Some clinicians also include as negative symptoms poverty of speech (extreme in mutism), and negative motor symptoms (catatonia, stupor, waxy flexibility, posturing). (*CTP 835. Har 269.*)

13. (4) Imaging techniques to study brain functions consist of computed axial tomography scanning (CAT scan) and magnetic resonance imaging (MRI). Both look at gross brain structures. Positive emission tomography (PET) and regional cerebral blood flow (RCBF) look at brain metabolism. Brain mapping (BEAM) compares the various areas of brain electrical activity.

In schizophrenia, imaging studies show ventricular enlargement as the most frequent and consistent finding with sulcal enlargement or cerebellar atrophy in 5–40% of cases. Schizophrenics are more likely to show a decrease in cerebral size, due to decrease of the frontal lobe, and cortical atrophy; these findings are not specific to schizophrenia as they are also seen in bipolar disorders. (*CTP 708-10. APA 383-85. Har 286-87.*)

14. (2) *Hypnogogic hallucinations* are false sensory perceptions that occur in the semiconscious state immediately preceding sleep and are of no pathological significance. (*CTP 474. APA 1254. Har 40.*)

15. (3) Drug induced psychotic syndromes can be seen in amphetamine psychosis (which has been considered as a model for paranoid schizophrenia) and reserpine depression (a model for unipolar depression). (*CTP 670-71.*)

16. (1) The essential features of paranoid personality disorder are a pervasive and unwarranted suspiciousness and mistrust of people. There is a tendency to be suspicious, mistrustful, hypervigilant, and preoccupied with perceived exploitation by others. Individuals with this syndrome do not have psychotic symptoms such as delusions. There may be a biogenic association with schizophrenia and paranoid disorder. Supportive psychotherapy may be the optimal therapy approach. Medications are usually ineffective or rejected by the patient. (*CTP 1365-67. APA 630-31. Har 342.*)

17. (3) In *factitious disorder*, there is the conscious, deliberate and surreptitious feigning of physical or psychological symptoms in order to simulate a disease. The individual goal is to be in the role of a patient. This disorder is in contrast to *malingering* where the goal is money, disability, or relief of work or military responsibility. Factitious disorder is similar to Munchausen's syndrome and pathological lying (pseudologica fantastica). Patients with factitious disorder often have a history of medical or nursing training. Symptoms include everything from infections, fever, chronic wounds, and self-medication to dermatologic and cardiac problems.

Treatment starts with suspecting the diagnosis and often requires collaboration with other physicians and a family evaluation. The patients will deny such behavior and generally will sign out AMA. Psychotherapy can be of some value if the patient is cooperative. (*CTP 1136-40. APA 549-52.*)

18. (4) Patients with personality disorders show patterns of inflexible and maladaptive behavior that cause significant impairments in social or occupational function, distress to others, or both. These disorders are not time-limited. The chronic maladaptive behavior patterns start early in life with an insidious onset and are usually evident by late adolescence or early adulthood. Individuals with a personality disorder are unable to respond in a flexible manner. They provoke aversive reactions in others and tend to blame others for problems. They do not have cognitive distortions. (*CTP 1352-53. APA 621. Har 338-41.*)

19. (2) The essential feature of *schizoid personality disorder* is the detachment from social relationships. These patients show a profound defect in the ability to form personal relationships or to respond to others in any meaningful, emotional way. They show an indifference to others by being aloof, detached, and unresponsive to praise, criticism, or feelings expressed by others. They tend to be solitary and preoccupied with their own inner

world, but they do not show cognitive distortions. Group therapy may be helpful for these patients, but few seek psychotherapy. (*CTP 1367-68. APA 629-30. Har 343-44.*)

20. (5) Patients with *narcissistic personality disorder* show expressions of grandiosity, entitlement, exploitation, emotional shallowness, and low empathy. They have a need for fame, wealth, or grand achievement and are preoccupied with beauty, strength, and youthful attributes. They tend to be hypersensitive to evaluation by others and react with shame, rage, humiliation, outward gross indifference or denial. Although conceited and arrogant, they are envious of others. The disorder begins in early adulthood.

Treatment ranges from intensive psychotherapy to brief therapy but abrupt termination is common. They are particularly prone to depressive and angry reactions when any threats occur to their self-esteem. Overall, they have less anxiety and chaotic reactions, fewer suicide attempts, and are less prone to psychotic decompensation than borderline personality disorder patients. (*CTP 1372-73. APA 632-34. Har 345-49.*)

21. (3) Defense mechanisms of the *borderline personality disorder* are fixated at the preoedipal phases of oral dependency and primitive aggression. These patients show difficulties in distinguishing fantasy from reality. They did not develop the capacity for basic trust. (*CTP 1377. APA 636-37. Har 232, 348.*)

22. (B) Eighty percent of patients with *panic disorders* or *agoraphobia* with panic attacks have anticipatory or generalized anxiety that is responsive to treatment with benzodiazepines, particularly alprazolam and clonazepam (but with a risk of dependence). For most patients, low doses of imipramine, desipramine, or nortriptyline should prove effective. Patients are initially very sensitive to the stimulant effects of antidepressants. MAOIs are reserved for those not responsive to heterocyclic antidepressants. (*APA 813-14. CTP 1584-85. Har 238.*)

23. (E) Panic attacks can be induced by drugs such as cocaine, marijuana, alcohol, sedatives, LSD, amphetamines, by hypothyroidism or hyperthyroidism, or by life events such as threatening illness or accidents, loss of a close personal relationship, or separation from family. Mitral valve prolapse may be associated with panic attacks. (*CTP 968. APA 444-45. Har 236-37.*)

24. (A) *Panic disorder* is usually seen in young adults, most often in the third decade, though some occur in the elderly. The morbidity risk among relatives of patients is 24.7% versus 2.3% for normal controls. Panic disorders are five times more frequent in monozygotic (80–90%) than dizygotic twins (10–15%). Fifteen to 17% of first-degree relatives are affected with panic, whereas 20%

have agoraphobia. Sex distribution of panic disorder without agoraphobia is equal, but panic disorder with agoraphobia is 2:1 female to male. (*CTP 952-55. APA 449. Har 449.*)

25. (E) *Conversion disorder* (hysterical neurosis, conversion type) can most readily be diagnosed when there is a temporal relationship between an emotional stressor and the initiation or exacerbation of the physical symptom. Symbolism, secondary gain, "la belle indifference," and histrionic traits may be present, but are not specific. The diagnosis is more frequent (2–5 times) in women than men. Conversion disorders occur in 5–13% of general hospital patients, with 30% also showing organic symptoms. A prolonged conversion symptom in the neuromuscular system may result in contractures. (*CTP 1013-17. APA 535-38. Har 250-54.*)

26. (E) In conversion disorder, there is some evidence of a family aggregation and a tendency to occur in the youngest child in the family. It is most common in adolescents and young adults, lower socioeconomic groups, rural populations, and those with less education. There is a basic conflict between instinctual impulse (aggressive or sexual) and the prohibitions against expression. (*CTP 1013-17. Har 253.*)

27. (D) Conversion reactions may be superimposed on organic seizures; therefore, EEG monitoring would be important. Patients with pseudoseizures can act wild or disorganized with theatrical thrashing that is a caricature of a true seizure. However, in contrast to a true seizure, they can recall events, rarely hurt themselves, or are usually not incontinent. It is always important to rule out an organic lesion. (*CTP 1013-17. APA 538.*)

28. (A) *Multiple personalities* is a most arresting form of dissociative hysteria. The true incidence and prevalence are unknown. The onset is in childhood, usually before age 9, and the majority of subjects are female, 75–90%. There is a frequent history of physical and sexual abuse in childhood (97–98%), especially in females. Multiple personality often occurs in several generations and with siblings. In this syndrome, two or more distinct identities are present within a single person, usually with amnesia for the altered or other personalities. (*CTP 1036-38. APA 570-72. Har 247-50.*)

29. (C) *Psychogenic fugue* is the major type of a dissociative disorder. It is reported most frequently in populations exposed to war, major psychosocial stress, and natural disasters. The patient suddenly and unexpectedly travels away from home or job, and cannot recall the past. There is an assumption of a new identity, which can be partial or complete during the fugue period of time. (*CTP 1035-36. APA 567. Har 246-70.*)

30. (C) In *psychogenic amnesia*, there is the sudden inability to recall important personal information that goes beyond ordinary forgetfulness. With psychogenic amnesia, memory returns completely, but in organic amnesia, memory does not return intact. Hypnosis or a short-acting barbiturate (thiopental and sodium amobarbital—Amytal) may be helpful in psychogenic memory recovery; in organic amnesia, barbiturate worsens symptoms and hypnosis may not be possible due to the individual's poor concentration ability.

    The duration of psychogenic amnesia is usually time-limited, whereas in organic amnesia, memory loss is chronic. The causes of psychogenic amnesia are primarily psychosocial stressors. In organic amnesia, the etiology ranges from trauma and substance intoxication to severe intracranial pathology. (*CTP 1034-35. APA 560-65, 569. Har 379-80.*)

31. (C) A *premenstrual syndrome* (PMS), or problems related to the menstrual cycle, occurs in 70–90% of women during the child-bearing ages. In the menstrual cycle, symptoms begin soon after ovulation and increase to maximum intensity about five days before the menstrual period. (*CTP 1218-19.*)

32. (E) *Anxiety disorder* and symptoms of anxiety can be seen in many medical conditions especially cardiovascular (mitral valve prolapse, myocardial infarction), pulmonary (asthma), neurologic (seizures), and endocrine (thyroid difficulties), and during drug intoxications (especially stimulants) and withdrawal (especially alcohol). (*CTP 968.*)

33. (E) A fear of leaving home may be due to anxiety, major depression, schizophrenia, paranoid personality disorder, avoidant personality disorder, or dependent personality disorder. (*APA 466. CTP 982.*)

34. (A) Treatment of an *obsessive compulsive disorder* (OCD) is most effective with psychopharmacotherapy, especially clomipramine (Anafranil). Phenelzine may be of value, and there are some newer drugs, fluvoxamine and fluoxetine (Prozac), that are stated to be effective. Supportive psychotherapy and, in some cases, analytic therapy may be beneficial. Behavior therapy is reported to be 60–70% successful, using desensitization, thought stopping, flooding, implosion therapy, aversive conditioning, and response prevention. Leukotomy has been used to treat incapacitating obsessive compulsive disorder. (*CTP 999. APA 478. Har 245.*)

35. (B) There is evidence that obsessive compulsive disorder (OCD) is associated with encephalitis epidemics, abnormal birth events, head injury, and seizures. First-degree relatives of OCD patients have increased depression and obsessional traits. There appears to be a genetic link between OCD and Tourette's disorder. Psychosocial factors relate to defenses of isolation, undoing, and reaction formation, with regression to the anal-sadistic phase, thereby allowing avoidance of genital conflicts and ambivalence. (*CTP 984-1000. APA 472-78. Har 241-44.*)

36. (B) The essential features of *post-traumatic stress disorder* (PTSD) are psychic numbing, reexperiencing of the trauma, and increased arousal. Long-term physical health effects were noted after 30 years in surviving concentration camp victims. Crisis intervention shortly after the traumatic event is effective in reducing immediate distress and possibly preventing chronic or delayed response.

    Treatment consists of tricyclic antidepressants, especially amitriptyline, imipramine, and phenelzine. Clonidine and propranolol also may be of some value. Antipsychotics are indicated with severe agitation. Psychotherapy, particularly group therapy and family and supportive groups, is helpful. (*APA 479-86. CTP 1000-1008. Har 245.*)

37. (E) *Generalized anxiety disorder* (GAD) is the chronic form of anxiety neurosis (anxiety states). The most common symptoms are:

    Motor tension—easy fatigability, restlessness, feeling shaky, trembling, inability to relax, easily startled
    Autonomic hyperactivity—tachycardia, palpitations, shortness of breath, dry mouth, sweating, urination, diarrhea, light-headedness
    Vigilance and scanning—trouble falling or staying asleep, insomnia, difficulty concentrating, irritability, impatience (*CTP 958-59. APA 446-47. Har 235-38.*)

38. (E) Major depressions are associated with sleep problems. The most common sleep abnormality in depression is insomnia, especially problems in remaining asleep rather than falling asleep. About 80–85% of patients demonstrate hyposomnia, whereas the rest experience hypersomnia. There is an abbreviated 1st NREM (short REM latency), and prolonged 1st REM with heightened density of REM. A large increase in early REM sleep occurs after sleep deprivation and decreased stage 4 sleep. (*APA 748. CTP 898. Har 160-61.*)

39. (B) *Melancholia* or *endogenous depression* has a positive correlation with age (older more likely to be endogenous, and younger reactive), and with personality (more likely in the relatively stable and nonneurotic). There is a negative correlation with life stresses and with a recent history of precipitating events. (*CTP 904. Har 318.*)

40. (B) Refer to question 2, Chapter 7, Community Psychiatry, reference postpartum psychosis. (*CTP 852-58, 1219.*)

41. **(A)** Depression occurs in 20–40% of medically ill patients. The following medical disorders can initially present as a depressive disorder:

    Endocrine: problems with thyroid, pituitary, and adrenal functioning
    Neurological: multiple sclerosis, Wilson's disease
    Collagen: systemic lupus erythematosus
    Nutritional/vitamins, minerals: pellagra, hypervitaminosis, beri-beri, pernicious anemia
    Infections: encephalitis, hepatitis, tuberculosis
    Cardiovascular: side effects of hypertensive medications, post-myocardial infarction
    Malignancies: anticancer medications, metastases
    Head trauma: concussion, especially subdural hematoma, encephalopathy.
    (See question 42 regarding medications and depression.) (*CTP 901. APA 416. Har 410.*)

42. **(A)** Medications that can cause depression:

    Corticosteroids—cortisone
    Anticancer drugs—vincristine, vinblastine
    Antituberculosis drugs—cycloserine
    Antiparkinson drugs—levodopa, carbidopa, amantadine
    Antihypertensives—reserpine, methyldopa, clonidine, propranolol
    Hormones—estrogens, progesterone (*CTP 901. APA 417. Har 734.*)

43. **(E)** About 50% of hospitalized patients with unipolar depressions (even lower in outpatients) have an abnormal or positive DST (a failure of dexamethasone to suppress cortisol secretion). A positive test is present when the post-dexamethasone serum cortisol level is equal to or exceeds 5 μg/dl. A false positive DST can be caused by weight loss, medications (steroids, estrogens, carbamazepine, indomethacin, barbiturates), diabetes, certain forms of schizophrenia, obsessive compulsive disorder, borderline personality disorder, and alcoholism. (*CTP 874. APA 265, 420, 523. Har 134-35.*)

44. **(B)** *Seasonal affective disorder* occurs as a depression in late fall or winter with a remission in spring progressing to hypomania in summer. It is an "atypical" depression, and there is a poor response to treatment by antidepressants. Treatment is with several hours of bright artificial light (sufficient to suppress plasma melatonin) of about 2,500 lux or 225 foot-candles. (*CTP 869, 1685-86. APA 433.*)

45. **(C)** Depressed patients have difficulty in sustaining self-esteem, related to feelings of helplessness. Learned helplessness is a theory of depression (Seligman), in which it is postulated that depression develops because of cognitive, emotional, and motivational deficiency, resulting in loss of control over events or experiences. (*APA 427. CTP 330-31. Har 313.*)

46. **(A)** Arnold Beck (1969) emphasized cognitive impairment among depressives, where the individuals have a decreased ability to assess their own performance and others' views of them. Cognitive theory states that depression results from the activation of specific cognitive distortions that are present in depression-prone people, called "depressogenic schemata." The stressor activates responses in these depression-prone subjects that leads to unrealistic negative and demeaning views of themselves, the world, and the future (referred to as the "cognitive triad"). (*APA 426-27. CTP 891. Har 313.*)

47. **(C)** A universal trend in affective disorders is the greater prevalence of depressive disorders among women (2:1 over men), especially with the unipolar disorders (4–5:1 over men). The difference is less marked with bipolar disorder where males about equal females. The lifetime expectancy for moderate to severe mood disorders is 8–10% for men and 16–20% for women. (*CTP 893. APA 82. Har 82.*)

48. **(A)** Disorders more common in women than men are affective (see question 47), anxiety, and somatization disorders. (*CTP 324. APA 84. Har 322.*)

49. **(C)** There is no clear-cut relationship existing between major depression and social class or race. However, rates of depression are highest in the unmarried and widowed groups, and within six months after a separation. Major depressions are more common than bipolar and more frequent in females (2:1). In major depressions, the age of onset is 20–50 years, whereas in bipolar disorder onset is in late adolescence to 30, with peak age in the 20s. (*APA 409-10. CTP 863-65. Har 321-22.*)

50. **(D)** General epidemiological data on lifetime prevalence. Major depressions: females 5–9%; in males 2–4% (2:1). Bipolar depression: males almost similar to females, 0.6–0.9%, (1:1.2). The family history is important in major depression. Major depression occurs in 17%, and bipolar depression in 2–3% of close relatives, whereas in relatives of bipolar patients, major depression occurs in 15%, and bipolar depression in 8%. (See questions number 47 and 49.) (*CTP 863-65. APA 410. Har 321-22.*)

51. **(E)** A manic episode may be induced by the use of antidepressant medication in bipolar patients. Psychosis, alcohol, drug abuse, suicide attempts, obsessive compulsive disorder, and encephalitis may produce mania symptoms in any patient. Drugs associated with causing manic behavior include stimulants, bromides, cocaine, cimetidine, disulfiram, hallucinogens, isoniazid, levodopa, opiates, and yohimbine. (*CTP 904-5.*)

52. **(B)** Lithium is the drug of choice for manic patients needing long-range treatment, but delusional, disruptive patients may initially require antipsychotics (phenothi-

azines, butyrophenones) or sedation using perhaps IM lorazepam, carbamazepine (Tegretol), L-tryptophan, ECT, valproic acid, clonidine, and clonazepam. (See question 8 reference rapid cycling patients.) (*CTP 924-26. Har 315.*)

53. **(E)** Patients require hospitalization if they are suicidal, have physical problems with weight and sleep, severe agitation, or need special diagnostic procedures. Electroconvulsive therapy (ECT) is the most effective treatment for unipolar depression manifested by nihilistic behavior and when a rapid therapeutic response is indicated. Amphetamines can be added to a heterocyclic antidepressant to increase effectiveness. Other treatments include MAOIs, supplemental L-triiodothyronine (T3), and antipsychotics. (*CTP 922-23. APA 429-30. Har 326-34.*)

54. **(E)** Highest rates of suicide are discussed in questions 9, 56, and 57. (*APA 1024. Har 744-45.*)

55. **(D)** The incidence of suicide is noted in question numbers 9 and 10. (*APA 1023-24. Har 744-45.*)

56. **(E)** There is an increased suicide risk in patients with a history of suicide attempts (10% who attempted suicide complete at a later time), a family history of suicide, depression (80% who commit suicide are said to be depressed), and who have communicated their suicidal intention to others (80% have told others). Seriously suicidal depressed patients commonly refuse to accept help and may have a definite resolve to die. Patients with severe physical illnesses also have an increased suicidal risk if they have a low tolerance for pain, make excessive demands or complaints, and perceive a lack of support from the medical staff. (*APA 1023-35. Har 744-45.*)

57. **(B)** Individuals who have made previous suicide attempts have a higher risk for subsequent suicide behavior. There are eight times more suicide attempts than successful suicides. About 70% of suicide attempts are made by women, mostly angry, frustrated, or depressed young adults. About 10% who attempt suicide eventually succeed, 30% make subsequent attempts, and the highest risk is within three months of first attempt.

Suicidal behavior may be coercive to others, a cry for help, or a gamble with death. Disorganized suicide attempts are usually made by disorganized, schizoid, or schizotypal patients. Successful suicide subjects are more likely to have had formulated a definite plan, made previous attempts, had previous suicidal thoughts, and talked to others about it. (Refer to answer in question 56.) (*CTP 1426. APA 1032. Har 744-45.*)

58. **(A)** The management of the suicidal patient is to hospitalize, either voluntarily or involuntarily. Suicidal behavior is a psychiatric emergency. Antidepressants can be used but can be dangerous since small amounts can be lethal; therefore these drugs should be dispensed in low amounts, and taken under close supervision. Electroconvulsive therapy (ECT) may be indicated. Outpatient follow-up is required. (Refer to question number 53.) (*CTP 1425. APA 1032-33. Har 326-34.*)

59. **(B)** *Hysteroid dysphoria* (Klein) is, in contrast to "endogenomorphic" depression, a reactive mood disorder with extreme fatigue, atypical vegetative symptoms, hypersomnia with initial insomnia, and hyperphagia. Sensitivity to rejection is a precipitating cause. Individuals are responsive to MAOIs. (*APA 406-7.*)

60. **(C)** Eugen Bleuler and Emil Kraepelin (1887) grouped psychotic conditions based on causal origin into those caused by external conditions and therefore curable, and others produced by inherent constitutional factors and therefore incurable. Bleuler renamed dementia praecox as schizophrenia and considered schizophrenia to be a group of disorders. He believed that the common abnormality in schizophrenics was cognitive impairment or thought disorder called "splitting," or "loosening" in the "fabric of thought." A group of symptoms were fundamental (4 A's—*Associations, Affect, Autism, Ambivalence*), whereas other symptoms such as delusions and hallucinations were considered *Accessory*. He further observed that some patients recover and others become chronic and that deterioration or dementia is not inevitable (as Kraepelin had thought). (*APA 358-59. Har 75.*)

61. **(E)** The *"dopamine hypothesis"* states that symptoms of schizophrenia are due to a hyperactivity in the dopamine system. This theory is based on the observation that drugs that block dopamine receptors (including resperine) are most effective in reducing the symptoms of schizophrenia. In addition, drugs that enhance dopamine transmission (amphetamine) tend to exacerbate the symptoms of schizophrenia. Most neuroleptics are more potent in the D2 receptor blockage. (*CTP 718-21. APA 382-83. Har 146-47.*)

62. **(C)** Genetic factors in schizophrenia:

Incidence 0.3/1,000
Prevalence 3.6/1,000 (lifetime prevalence 1–1.9%)
Mean age, men develop earlier (21.4 years) than women (26.8 years)
Children, where both parents are schizophrenic, have a 10% lifetime risk
Children, where one parent is schizophrenic, have a 5–6% lifetime risk
Increased risk of 17–46% when more than two first-degree family members have schizophrenia
Monozygotic twins have a 46% concordance rate compared with 14% for dizygotic twins
(*CTP 702. APA 375-79. Har 139-42.*)

63. **(C)** Schizophrenia in males is diagnosed earlier than in females. Schizophrenics have, on the average, a lower class standing, referred to as a manifestation of the "drift hypothesis" (Wender 1973). More live in slum areas than in suburban areas. This is a culturally universal phenomenon. (See question number 62.) (*CTP 701-4. APA 382. Har 140-42.*)

64. **(B)** *Paranoid schizophrenia*, compared with other subtypes, is less likely to have an age of onset before age 25. These patients are more likely to be married, have children, and be employed. Relatives of schizophrenics have higher risk for schizophrenia than those without schizophrenic relatives. Paranoid schizophrenics have one or more systematized delusions or frequent auditory hallucinations related to a single theme, with flat or inappropriate affect or bizarre behavior in the absence of a florid thought disorder. (*CTP 770. APA 371. Har 283.*)

65. **(B)** The cardinal feature of the *delusional* (paranoid) *disorder* is the delusion (false belief) maintained in the face of contradictory evidence and not shared by others. The disorder is unrelated to schizophrenia or affective disorder. The delusions are not flagrantly bizarre, and auditory or visual hallucinations are not prominent. With this syndrome, males have a greater rate than females, generally the age of incidence is 20–40 years old, and these patients usually have a satisfactory work history. (*CTP 816-29. APA 393. Har 296-307.*)

66. **(E)** Stupor, mutism, rigidity, and negativism are not specific to one disorder, and can be symptoms in a number of syndromes, from substance abuse, toxic reactions (neuroleptics), medical problems (especially parkinsonism or encephalitis), to mental illness (such as depression, schizophrenia, and post-traumatic stress disorder). (*APA 365-66. CTP 457.*)

67. **(C)** Patients with *schizoaffective disorder*, unlike schizophrenia, have a good premorbid adjustment, an acute onset, a remitting course, and more often a good recovery. Schizoaffective disorder usually begins in the early 20s with no difference in sex distribution. Some consider this syndrome to be an affective disorder, others a variant of schizophrenia, and still others an independent syndrome. (*CTP 830-37. APA 415-16. Har 320.*)

68. **(C)** The family is the real treatment team most of the time when working with schizophrenics. A psychoeducational model is necessary in working with these patients and their families. Family members should be educated concerning the illness and medication, and helped to reduce their guilt and self-blame for the patient's illness. Lowering expectations to a level of solving daily household problems and then working up to more complex matters is the basic rehabilitation method. Families can be more helpful to the patient by not being intrusive and

thereby not provoking potentially disruptive anxiety. (*CTP 792-806. APA 942-49. Har 276.*)

69. **(A)** The prognosis for the schizophrenic patient is better when there are affective components to the symptoms and less intellectual deterioration (as seen with paranoid schizophrenia). Other good prognostic features are a beneficial response to medications, being a female, less institutional care, an acute onset, confusion, short duration of an episode, no prior psychiatric history, steady work history, married, older age of onset, normal neurologic function, negative family history, high social class, and normal CAT scan.

A regression analysis revealed five most powerful predictors for a poor prognosis—social isolation, long duration of episode, past psychiatric treatment, unmarried, and behavior problems in childhood such as truancy and tantrums. Other factors for a poor prognosis are structural brain abnormalities, obsessive compulsive symptoms, assaultiveness, affective blunting, long duration, and an insidious onset. (*CTP 768. APA 369-70. Har 277-79.*)

70. **(A)** The *intermittent explosive disorder* is different from any other personality disorder. Of all the violent disorders, it has the best prognosis. The disorder is manifested by discrete episodes of loss of control involving violence toward others or destruction of property. The violence is out of proportion to any precipitating factors, usually directed toward family members, often in a marital relationship and frequently associated with alcohol use. The episode is followed by remorse and feelings of guilt. Between episodes there are few problems with control or violence. There is usually a past childhood history of an unfavorable environment, alcoholism, beatings, threats to life, and promiscuity. Patients usually report a poor work history with marital difficulties and trouble with the law. (*CTP 1152-53. APA 1043.*)

71. **(E)** *Antisocial personality disorder* is more frequent in males (4–7 times greater than in females) and is more prevalent in urban areas. The peak prevalence occurs during ages 24–44, then drops off after age 45. Family and twin studies have demonstrated some degree of biogenetic and environmental predispositions to antisocial and criminal behavior. There is a familial association with histrionic personality disorder. Before age 15, many patients manifest problems with truancy, running away, lying, stealing, and physical cruelty.

Individuals with this disorder seem to have a reduced level of inhibitory anxiety, which contributes to the impulsive, sensation-seeking lifestyle, and a failure to be responsive to aversive consequences. There may be an association among attention deficit hyperactivity disorder and early abnormalities in the prenatal and perinatal period and later antisocial behavior, but this is still unclear. (*CTP 1374-75. APA 634-36. Har 346-47.*)

72. **(A)** Antisocial personality disorder is one of the most difficult personality disorders to treat. These subjects have a lack of empathy and social responsibility and a tendency to try to outwit the therapist rather than effect a positive change. A correctional facility or a residential treatment program may be the only means of controlling the individual and attempting to produce a change of behavior. Marital and family therapy may be helpful as well as confrontational groups with other antisocial personality disorder patients. Behavior therapy may be useful in a highly structured environment. Medications are nonspecific and may be abused, but lithium or propranolol may be useful for violent episodes. (*CTP 1373-77. APA 634-36. Har 346-47.*)

73. **(B)** *Pathological gambling* is seen in the risk-taker who fails to profit from his or her gambling misadventure. These subjects are unable to stop when winning. Pathological gambling is closely associated with drinking. Individuals resent intrusion of any authority figures. Most pathological gamblers are likely to be married and have provided reasonably for the family before the gambling losses started. Rarely does a pathological gambler seek psychiatric help. It is estimated that they make up 2–3% of the adult population.

 Pathological gambling and alcoholism are more common in fathers of males and mothers of females. Inconsistent parental discipline, exposure to gambling as an adolescent, and a family that places high value on material symbols and low emphasis on savings and budgets are common background factors. Relapses are common. Individuals have a high incidence of major affective disorders with a high risk for suicide. Gamblers Anonymous (GA), Gam-Anon (for family and spouses), Gam-a-Teen (for adolescents and children), and self-help programs may be helpful. The outcome is similar to that of alcoholism self-help groups. (*CTP 1146-47. APA 613-16.*)

74. **(E)** The essential feature of *self-defeating personality disorder* is the repetitive patterns of continuing with avoidable, self-defeating behavior and relationships, despite complaining of being victimized. It is similar to the "masochistic," "self-effacing," or "depressive" personality disorders.

 Individuals show chronic pessimism, submissive and acquiescent attitudes, a resignation to failure, and a tendency to place themselves in situations and relationships that are harmful, painful, disappointing, or abusive. These patients are difficult to treat and they expect treatment to fail. Therapist countertransference problems are common because these individuals incite anger or rejection and reject the opportunity for pleasure. Adjunctive marital or family treatment will often be needed. Depression may have to be treated; otherwise there are no specific medications for patients with this syndrome. (*APA 643-44. CTP 1385-88. Har 354-55.*)

75. **(D)** *Malingering* is the intentional production of physical or psychological symptoms motivated by external incentives (avoiding work, military duty, financial responsibilities; obtaining drugs). It may be difficult to differentiate between factitious disorder and malingering if the goal is drug-seeking. It is a V code reference "not attributable to a mental disorder." The various types of malingering are: (1) the staged event, (2) data tampering, (3) opportunistic, (4) symptom invention, (5) self-destructive behavior. (See question number 17 reference factitious disorder.) (*APA 553-54. CTP 1396-99. Har 100.*)

76. **(C)** *Type A personality* characteristics usually include competitiveness, time urgency, aggression, impatience, and frequently a lack of pleasure manifested by abrupt gestures and explosive speech. These subjects also show high levels of impatience, frustration, anger and hostility, competitiveness, and constant striving for signs of success. This type of behavior is seen in many coronary heart disease and myocardial infarction patients.

 Type B personality is the opposite of Type A, and is described as not having these traits. Some report that Type A individuals have two times the coronary heart disease as Type B individuals. Anger and hostility are most strongly correlated with coronary heart disease, cancer, and death rates. "Holding in" frustrations and rapid explosive speech are also factors. MMPI shows high hostility scores. (*APA 498-501. CTP 1192-94. Har 398.*)

77. **(B)** The essential features of *passive aggressive personality disorder* are passive resistance and covert noncompliance with ordinary demands of social and occupational requirements. These patients tend to be passively and indirectly resistant to authority demands, obligations, and responsibilities, manifested by dawdling, procrastinating, and forgetting. They tend to complain, and are irritable, whining, argumentative, critical, discontented, disillusioned, and disgruntled. The individuals are difficult to treat but paradoxical technique and approaches may be effective. (*APA 641-42. CTP 1384. Har 353-54.*)

78. **(D)** *Borderline personality disorder* cuts across existing diagnostic categories. In these patients there is identity diffusion and primitive defense mechanisms (especially splitting). Frustrations result in overwhelming rage. Common features of the disorder include intense and chaotic relationships, with affective instability; fluctuating and extreme attitudes regarding other people; impulsive and self-destructive behavior; and a lack of clear or certain sense of identity, life plan, or values. Fear of real or imagined abandonment is a frequent preoccupation.

 A biogenic association with affective disorders appears likely, and the disorder is considered by some as a subaffective disorder based on family history, pharmacologic research, and follow-up. Borderline, histrionic, and schizotypal personality disorders overlap in many areas. (*CTP 1377-79. APA 636-37. Har 347-48.*)

79. **(E)** Psychotherapy with the borderline personality disorder patient consists of an intensive, interpretive, and confrontational psychotherapy, with a focus on transferential relationships. The patient commonly terminates prematurely. Group and marital therapy may be used to reduce the transference. Cognitive techniques may be helpful because of the patient's extreme attitudes and continued attempts at splitting the treatment team. Self-mutilation behavior and impulsive regressions are common.

Medications used include lithium, antidepressants (MAOIs), antipsychotics, minor tranquilizers (particularly alprazolam—Xanax), and carbamazepine (Tegretol). (See question number 78.) (*CTP 1377-79. APA 636-37. Har 347-48.*)

80. **(C)** Of all the personality disorders, borderline patients present the most varied and unstable behaviors and symptoms. (Refer to questions 78 and 79 for more details on the borderline personality disorder.) (*CTP 1377-79. APA 636-37. Har 347-48.*)

4

SPECIAL TOPICS
Geriatrics, Psychosexual Disorders, Eating Disorders, Sleep Disorders, and Somatopsychic Disorders

1. Increased risk of suicide in the elderly is associated with all of the following except:

   1. Divorce
   2. Alcoholism
   3. Male
   4. Chronic illness
   5. Minority group

2. When elderly adults are compared with young adults, all of the following statements are correct except:

   1. Increased cognitive impairment due to anticholinergics
   2. Increased risk of dystonic reactions with neuroleptics
   3. Increased risk of lithium toxicity due to longer half-life
   4. Increased risk of confusion and ataxia with diazepam
   5. Increased risk of post ECT delirium

3. All of the following statements about the elderly are correct except:

   1. Over age 65, the suicide rate for males is more than five times the female rate
   2. After age 65, about 25% stay in nursing homes or institutions
   3. The family is the primary caretaker of the elderly in the United States
   4. People who retire late tend to live longer
   5. Individual psychotherapy is therapeutically effective in the elderly

4. As part of normal aging, all of the following occur except:

   1. Decreased percentage of REM sleep
   2. Decreased percentage of stage 4 sleep
   3. Decreased glomerular filteration rate
   4. Increased gastric acid secretion
   5. Increased body fat relative to body mass

5. Which antidepressant would be indicated in the treatment of a depressed 70-year-old man with benign prostatic hypertrophy, arthritis of the right hip joint, and left bundle branch block?

   1. Amitriptyline
   2. Bupropion
   3. Trazodone
   4. Doxepin
   5. Desipramine

6. The most common cause for male erectile disorder is:

   1. Multiple sclerosis
   2. Spinal cord injury
   3. Prostatectomy
   4. Aortic vascular disease
   5. Diabetes mellitus

7. All of the following statements regarding transvestism are true except:

   1. Cross-dressing to produce sexual excitement
   2. Usually male with stable male identity
   3. Sexual preference is usually homosexual
   4. May show feminine behavior while cross-dressed
   5. Increased incidence of pedophilia

8. All of the following statements about anorexia nervosa are correct except:

   1. Better prognosis with late age of onset
   2. Dexamethasone nonsuppression
   3. Increased family incidence
   4. Increased risk of suicide
   5. More common in people who exercise frequently

9. All of the following symptoms are likely to occur in anorexia nervosa except:

1. Bradycardia
2. Leucopenia
3. Decreased body hair
4. Hypothermia
5. Cardiac arrhythmias

10. All of the following statements about REM sleep are correct except:

   1. REM sleep percentage is increased in chronic alcoholism
   2. REM latency under 70 minutes in patients with unipolar depression
   3. Caffeine before bedtime shifts REM sleep to the first half of the sleep cycle
   4. Withdrawal from chronic barbiturate use leads to REM
   5. Tricyclic antidepressants cause REM suppression

11. All of the following statements about patients with sleep apnea are correct except:

   1. Predominantly male
   2. Usually obese
   3. Bed partners complain of snoring
   4. Coexisting cardiac arrhythmias
   5. Episodic breathing difficulties during the day

12. All of the following statements about normal sleep patterns are correct except:

   1. Elderly tend to fall asleep earlier and waken earlier
   2. In the elderly, increase in number and duration of wakenings
   3. In young adults, most REM sleep occurs in the first half of the night
   4. Males have higher incidence of nocturnal myoclonus
   5. Young adult averages four to six sleep cycles per night

13. Appropriate management of sleep apnea could include all of the following except:

   1. ENT consultation
   2. Weight reduction programs
   3. Low dose flurazepam before bedtime
   4. Tracheostomy
   5. Nasal oxygen

14. All of the following statements about the restless legs syndrome are valid except:

   1. Disagreeable sensations within the calves
   2. Frequent during pregnancy
   3. Manifestation of generalized anxiety or depression
   4. Frequently get up to obtain relief
   5. Usually bilateral and symmetrical

15. All of the following statements about sleep terrors are accurate except:

1. Agitated, sweating, rapid breathing
2. Most often in the first half of night sleep
3. Most frequent age 5–12
4. Usually indicates underlying separation anxiety
5. Usually does not recall the episode next morning

16. Symptoms of narcolepsy include all of the following except:

   1. Hypnagogic hallucinations
   2. Cataleptic episodes precipitated by intense emotions
   3. Irresistible daytime sleep attacks
   4. Sleep paralysis
   5. Focal weakness of muscle groups

17. All of the following statements about acute intermittent porphyria are true except:

   1. Anxious, depressed, confused
   2. Symptoms precipitated or worsened by barbiturates
   3. May present with weakness in the legs
   4. Sweating, tachycardia, labile hypertension
   5. Typically males in late teens and early 20s

18. As part of a treatment plan for a patient with chronic pain, all of the following are appropriate except:

   1. Tricyclic antidepressant
   2. Hypnosis
   3. Benzodiazepines
   4. Nerve blocking
   5. Biofeedback

19. Predisposing factors to postoperative delirium include all of the following except:

   1. Preoperative anxiety
   2. Substance abuse
   3. Schizophrenia
   4. Preoperative organic brain disease
   5. Preoperative denial

20. All of the following statements about hemodialysis patients are correct except:

   1. Denial is not helpful to the patient
   2. Liable to intracranial bleeding
   3. Very high suicide rate
   4. High brain aluminum associated with dementia
   5. Sexual dysfunction common

21. All of the following are characteristic of adult onset hypothyroidism except:

   1. Depression and apathy common
   2. Mental slowing and cognitive impairment
   3. During initial thyroid replacement, psychiatric symptoms may worsen

4. Gradual thyroid replacement therapy causes mental symptoms to clear
5. Most common cause is autoimmune thyroiditis

22. All of the following are characteristic of delirium except:

    1. Onset over hours or a few days
    2. Varying arousal state
    3. Disturbance of sleep-wake cycle
    4. Absence of dementia
    5. Memory impairment

23. All of the following statements about placebo responses are correct except:

    1. One-third of patients with pain have definite relief with placebo
    2. Placebo does not cause physical side effects
    3. Placebo effect of analgesic is enhanced by giving a larger initial dose
    4. Patients have pain-relieving placebo effect regardless of the type of lesion
    5. Placebo effect may be blocked by morphine antagonists

24. All of the following statements about multiple sclerosis are correct except:

    1. More common in women
    2. Onset usually age 20 to 40
    3. More often in Mediterranean area people
    4. May cause syndrome similar to la belle indifference
    5. Unpredictable remissions

25. All of the following statements about hyperventilation episodes are valid except:

    1. Over-breathing causes carbon dioxide loss
    2. May develop tetanic flexures of the wrist
    3. Increased serum calcium
    4. Treated by breathing into a paper bag
    5. May over-breathe at normal rate

26. All of the following are aspects of normal grieving except:

    1. Feelings of anger toward medical or nursing personnel
    2. Feelings of failure and low self-worth
    3. Repeatedly remembering the deceased
    4. Feeling that the dead person is physically present
    5. Sadness and weeping openly manifest

27. In considering the five stages of dying as described by Kubler-Ross, which of the following statements is most accurate?

    1. Many patients do not move beyond the first stage of shock and denial
    2. Most patients pass through all five phases within two to three months

3. Most patients pass through all stages but in varying sequence
4. These stages are not unique to dying and are seen in response to other losses
5. The five stages are only present in the emotionally mature elderly patient

DIRECTIONS: For questions 28 through 83, one or more of the answers or completions given are correct. After you decide which alternatives are correct, record your answer according to the following key.

A if alternatives 1, 2 and 3 only are correct.
B if alternatives 1 and 3 only are correct.
C if alternatives 2 and 4 only are correct.
D if alternative 4 only is correct.
E if all four alternatives are correct.

28. When elderly subjects are compared with young adults, the elderly are likely to score lower on which of the following psychological tests?

    1. Vocabulary
    2. Visuo-spatial functions
    3. General information
    4. Timed tasks

29. Which of the following are normal concomitants of aging?

    1. Reduced ability to discriminate yellow from white
    2. Decreased parotid gland secretion
    3. Decreased hepatic oxidative ability
    4. 15% decrease in brain weight by age 80

30. Which of the following statements are correct about patients with AIDS-related complex?

    1. Tend to be more anxious and depressed than patients with AIDS
    2. Higher incidence of aseptic meningitis than in AIDS patients
    3. Frequently show evidence of cognitive impairment on screening neuropsychological testing
    4. Psychological responses similar to those seen in cancer patients

31. Which of the following statements regarding human immunodeficiency virus infection are correct?

    1. Early development of detectable antibodies protects against disease development
    2. Hemophiliac patients show more rapid disease progression
    3. HIV infection is not transmitted by breast milk
    4. HIV seropositive patients should be considered potentially infectious lifelong

32. Patients with AIDS dementia complex are likely to show which of the following?

    1. Elevated cerebrospinal fluid protein
    2. Generalized slowing on the electroencephalogram
    3. Cortical atrophy and ventricular enlargement on CT scan
    4. Reduced density of central white matter on MRI scan

33. Which of the following statements regarding the use of benzodiazepines in the elderly are correct?

    1. Diazepam tends to accumulate, causing confusion and ataxia
    2. Lorazepam does not cause amnesia
    3. Oxazepam may produce rebound daytime anxiety
    4. Oxazepam is very rapidly absolved orally

34. In the elderly, which of the following may cause symptoms of confusion?

    1. Depression
    2. Chlordiazepoxide
    3. Urinary tract infection
    4. Diuretics

35. Which of the following statements about dementia are correct?

    1. Disorder of thinking
    2. Invariably progressive
    3. Physical etiology
    4. Clouding of consciousness

36. Which of the following statements about multi-infarct dementia are accurate?

    1. Onset tends to be acute
    2. Focal neurological signs
    3. Stepwise deterioration
    4. More common in women

37. In a patient showing memory or orientation defects, which of the following would suggest depression rather than dementia as the primary cause?

    1. Very upset by the symptoms
    2. Does not try hard to perform with testing
    3. Complaints exceed demonstrated deficits
    4. Memory improves after electroconvulsive therapy

38. Changes in drug pharmacokinetics due to aging include:

    1. Increased ratio of adipose tissue to lean
    2. Hepatic glucuronide conjugation shows greater reduction than oxidative metabolism reduction
    3. Reduced renal clearance of lithium
    4. Increased total body water

39. Which of the following statements about lithium maintenance treatment in patients over age 60 are correct?

    1. Increased risk of toxicity with thiazide diuretics
    2. Lithium half-life increased in the elderly
    3. Steady-state levels take longer to achieve
    4. Hepatic clearance of lithium is slowed

40. When antidepressants are used with the elderly, which of the following statements are correct?

    1. When used for nighttime sedation, tend to accumulate
    2. Constipation may lead to noncompliance
    3. Percentage of antidepressant that is unbound in the plasma is increased
    4. Monoamine oxidase inhibitors are indicated when orthostatic hypotension is a problem

41. Which of the following statements about premature ejaculation are correct?

    1. More common in college educated
    2. Yohimbine therapeutic
    3. Treated with the stop-start technique
    4. Goal is to satisfy partner with each episode of coitus

42. In a physically healthy, young adult woman, not pregnant, amenorrhea may be caused by:

    1. Electroconvulsive therapy
    2. Haloperidol
    3. Pseudocyesis
    4. Lithium

43. In REM penile erection studies of adult males, which of the following statements are correct?

    1. Absence of erections indicates organic cause is 85% correct
    2. Depressed males may show absence of erections
    3. Males with vascular disease may have nocturnal erections but also organic-based impotence
    4. Determines whether medication is cause of impotence

44. Impotence in a 60-year-old male may be caused by which of the following factors acting together?

    1. Performance anxiety
    2. Lack of sexual partner
    3. Alcoholic cirrhosis
    4. Diabetes mellitus

45. Drugs that impair erectile function include:

    1. Fluphenazine
    2. Heroin
    3. Alcohol
    4. Reserpine

46. Which of the following statements about pedophilia are correct?

1. Pedophiles molesting boys show high recidivism
2. Pedophile victims are female twice as often as male
3. Vaginal penetration occurs usually only in incest
4. Pedophiles infrequently are exhibitionists

47. When homosexual rape is compared with heterosexual rape, which of the following statements are correct?

    1. Homosexual rape victims are more commonly male
    2. Dynamics are the same in homosexual and heterosexual rape
    3. Homosexual rape victims often fear becoming homosexual
    4. Both are highly unreported

48. In treating male pedophiles, which of the following statements are true?

    1. Early onset pedophilia has poorer prognosis
    2. Frequent pedophilia has poorer prognosis
    3. Alcoholic pedophilia has poorer prognosis
    4. Pedophilia with other sexual interest has poorer prognosis

49. In the inpatient management of anorexia nervosa patients, which of the following are appropriate?

    1. Bingeing patients to remain in public day room three hours after each meal
    2. Social activities permitted depending on meals finished
    3. Visiting privileges contingent on weight gain
    4. Patients should be encouraged to ignore weight status

50. When anorexia nervosa patients who binge and purge are compared with anorexia nervosa patients who only fast, the binge-purgers have which of the following characteristics?

    1. Higher incidence of drug abuse
    2. Lower incidence of suicide attempts
    3. More likely to be sexually active
    4. Younger age of onset

51. Which of the following statements about obesity in the United States are correct?

    1. More common in lower socioeconomic groups
    2. Obese parents tend to have obese children
    3. Obese children are likely to become obese adults
    4. Obese people have larger and more fat cells

52. In the treatment of moderate stable obesity, which of the following are important?

    1. Patient's motivation for weight loss
    2. Increased awareness of eating
    3. Cognitive restructuring
    4. Gradually increasing exercise

53. When gastrointestinal bypass surgery is compared with dieting in the treatment of morbid obesity, which of the following statements are valid?

    1. Increased incidence of divorce in postsurgery patients
    2. Greater incidence of anxiety and depression in postsurgery patients
    3. Increased emotional fluctuation in postsurgery patients
    4. Dieting patients have more positive body image

54. Patients with bulimia nervosa are more likely to have which of the following symptoms?

    1. Depression
    2. Suicidal behavior
    3. Diuretic abuse
    4. Kleptomania

55. Patients with bulimia nervosa are likely to show which of the following symptoms?

    1. Submandibular gland enlargement
    2. Erosion of dental enamel
    3. Esophageal tears
    4. Cardiac myopathy

56. Symptoms often seen in patients with anorexia nervosa include:

    1. Laxative abuse
    2. Excessive exercising
    3. Amenorrhea
    4. Kleptomania

57. When a patient drinks several cups of regular coffee shortly before going to bed, which of the following effects are likely to occur?

    1. Increased REM percentage
    2. REM sleep moved to latter half of night
    3. Decreased sleep latency
    4. Decrease total slow-wave sleep

58. Symptoms of sleep apnea are likely to include which of the following?

    1. Falling asleep during daytime
    2. Loud, continuous snoring during sleep
    3. Frequent associated hypertension
    4. Subject rises and paces the floor during arousal periods

59. Which of the following symptoms may be presenting manifestations of the sleep apnea syndrome?

    1. Poor job performance
    2. Personality changes
    3. Repeated driving accidents
    4. Impotence or decreased libido

60. Generally useful treatment for insomnia is likely to include:

1. A little brandy or whiskey just before bedtime
2. Reading or watching television in bed to relax before sleeping
3. A good brisk walk prior to retiring for bed
4. Establishing regular schedule for going to bed

61. Which of the following statements about sleep are correct?

1. Short sleepers may sleep less than people with insomnia, yet still feel rested
2. Depressed patients overestimate sleep latency and underestimate actual sleep
3. Effective treatment of depression corrects associated sleep disturbance
4. Elderly people tend to overestimate their need for sleep

62. Which of the following sleep study results are found in patients with unipolar depression?

1. Decreased sleep latency
2. Shortened REM latency
3. Decreased REM density
4. Reduced stage 4 sleep

63. Which of the following disorders may be diagnosed on polysomnographic examination?

1. Narcolepsy
2. Nocturnal myoclonus
3. Sleep apnea
4. Myasthenia gravis

64. Which of the following statements regarding sleep patterns of manic patients are correct?

1. Reduction in stage 3–4 sleep
2. Total sleep time shortened
3. Severe sleep onset insomnia
4. Frequent complaints of insomnia

65. Which of the following sleep disorders are more common among family members similarly affected?

1. Narcolepsy
2. Sleep paralysis
3. Sleepwalking
4. Bruxism

66. Which of the following statements regarding myoclonic sleep disorder are correct?

1. Patient may complain of insomnia or of excessive daytime sleepiness
2. Most common in middle-aged women
3. Anterior tibialis muscle periodic activity
4. Tricyclic antidepressants relieve symptoms

67. Normal sleep changes with aging include:

1. Total sleep time reduced
2. Total REM time increases
3. Stage 4 sleep may be absent
4. REM sleep occurs increasingly late in sleep

68. Which of the following statements about narcolepsy are correct?

1. Marked familial incidence
2. Most often in young males
3. Methylphenidate gives symptomatic improvement
4. Periods of confusion and excessive eating

69. In chronic alcoholics which of the following effects are likely to occur?

1. Total sleep time increased
2. REM sleep is fragmented
3. REM percentage is increased
4. During withdrawal from alcohol, slow-wave sleep decreases

70. Which of the following procedures would be appropriate management with a chronic pain patient?

1. Adequate analgesic prescribed on an as-needed basis
2. Referral to a specialized inpatient unit
3. Placebo to differentiate organic from psychogenic pain
4. Regular scheduled physician contact

71. In planning the management of a patient after a myocardial infarction, which of the following statements are correct?

1. Depression is almost universal at some time in the first month
2. Weakness can be expected as a manifestation of cardiac inefficiency
3. Coitus can be resumed one month after infarction
4. Anxiolytics should be prescribed on as-needed basis

72. In management of the anxious, depressed patient with chronic obstructive pulmonary disease, which of the following apply?

1. Chronic hypoxia decreased cognitive efficiency
2. Amitriptyline at bedtime is often beneficial
3. Any increase in emotion worsens dyspnea
4. Propranolol worsens bronchospasm

73. Psychiatric syndromes often associated with Parkinson's disease include:

1. Depression
2. Agoraphobia
3. Dementia
4. Panic disorder

74. In management of systemic lupus erythematosus, which of the following statements are correct?

    1. Exacerbation may cause confusion
    2. Thought disorder may mimic schizophrenia
    3. Predominantly females affected
    4. Toxic psychosis frequently due to steroid overdose

75. Which of the following statements apply to both delirium and dementia?

    1. Memory disturbance
    2. Disorder of thinking
    3. Organic etiology
    4. Clouding of consciousness

76. Which of the following statements regarding delirium are correct?

    1. 20% of delirious patients present with depression and anxiety
    2. 20% of delirious patients present with delusions and hallucinations
    3. 20% of delirious patients present with demanding, uncooperative behavior
    4. 30% of delirious patients present with confusion and disorientation

77. The management of delirium of unknown cause should include which of the following?

    1. Transfer to a psychiatric unit
    2. Keep the environment as quiet as possible
    3. Alprazolam six hourly
    4. Low-dose haloperidol

78. The risk of delirium is increased in which of the following groups?

    1. Elderly over age 60
    2. Children before age 5
    3. Chronic alcoholics
    4. Patients receiving ulcer medication

79. An organic mood disorder may be caused by:

    1. Multiple sclerosis
    2. Infectious mononucleosis
    3. L-dopa
    4. Propranolol

80. Patients after vasectomy are likely to show which of the following?

    1. Reactive depression
    2. Reduced sexual drive
    3. Impotency
    4. Increased sexual potency

81. Which of the following about hyperventilation are correct?

    1. Caused by salicylate toxicity

    2. Produced by brainstem infection
    3. Manifestation of diabetic acidosis
    4. Dose-related reserpine effect

82. Which of the following statements describe the usual course of a patient with myocardial infarction?

    1. Immediate strong denial, gradually lessening after 1–2 days
    2. Depression starts after 3–4 days and persists after hospital discharge
    3. Constant cardiac monitoring is felt as a constant stressing factor
    4. Anxiety is maximal in the first 1–2 days after the attack, and is then followed by denial

83. Following myocardial infarction, which of the following statements are correct?

    1. Anxiety raises catecholamines with risk of arrhythmias
    2. Anxiety is raised by leaving the hospital
    3. Moderate denial improves the prognosis
    4. Cardiac monitor is a constant cause of anxiety

ANSWERS AND EXPLANATIONS

1. (5) There is a higher incidence of suicide in the elderly (over 65 years) who make up 10–11% of the population but 17–25% of all suicides. Loss is the predominant theme in suicide of the elderly. Depression may mimic senile dementia so that suicide potential may be overlooked. Characteristics of successful suicides in the elderly are a white male with a combination of psychiatric problems (persistence of depression into old age), chronic physical and medical illnesses, retirement, loss of a spouse, and loneliness.

   The suicide rate is greater in elderly males despite the fact that there are more elderly women living than males. Elderly white males have a 10–30 times greater incidence of suicide than elderly white females, whereas elderly black males have a 4–6 times higher rate than elderly black females. (*CTP 1414-24. APA 1023, 1031. Har 671.*)

2. (2) Most biological changes during old age are gradual and progressive including changes in nerve conduction time, heart rate, blood pressure, and increased tremors. Toxins of bacterial and metabolic origin are common, resulting in physical and mental problems. Cerebral anoxia can occur from cardiac or respiratory disease. Alzheimer's disease is present in 50% of patients in nursing homes. Although psychiatric illnesses are common in the elderly, they may be manifested primarily by physical symptoms and signs such as a loss of weight, constipation, and dry mouth.

   Many drugs can cause psychiatric symptoms in the elderly, especially with larger doses. The aged often need more frequent dosing because they cannot tolerate sudden rises in blood levels. Liquid forms of medication may be needed due to an inability or refusal to swallow. Toxic confusional states can result from the anticholinergic properties of many medications, especially the antipsychotics and tricyclics.

   Depressions initially starting in old age are most common in those individuals who have had a previous well-adjusted personality. Schizophrenia, manic disorder, neurosis, and anxiety disorder do not frequently start in old age. Hypochondriasis is very common, but obsessive compulsive disorder has about the same rate as in younger subjects. Sleep disturbances are common. (*CTP 2040-46. APA 1117-39. Har 665-67.*)

3. (2) Psychotherapy with the elderly has similar indications and effectiveness as with any age level. More than half of the elderly are physically unimpeded in their bodily movements, with 80% being able to perform all major daily tasks without help from another person, 95% are still living in the community, and 90% are still intellectually intact. Two-thirds live with someone else in the household, and 80% have a family member or friend who is willing to help look after them. (*CTP 2014. APA 1023, 1136-37. Har 666-67.*)

4. (4) In the aging process, there is a progressive decline in many body functions, especially decreases in cardiac output and stroke volume, glomerular filtration rate, oxygen consumption, cerebral blood flow, and vital capacity. A thickening of the optic lens occurs as well as a progressive hearing loss, particularly in the higher frequencies. The immune system is altered with impaired T-cell response, resulting in an increased susceptibility to infection and neoplasms.

   Anatomic changes include decrease in height and muscle mass, a deepening of thoracic cage, graying of the hair, and lengthening of the nose and ears. Osteoporosis and osteoarthritis are common. Changes in body weight are usually due to an increase in body fat. The heart may increase in size and weight.

   Endocrine functions change with a decrease in estrogens and testosterone but an increase in follicle stimulating hormone and luteinizing hormone. Within the CNS there is a decrease in brain weight, ventricular enlargement and neuronal loss, and a reduction in cerebral blood flow. Both NREM and REM sleep decrease with increasing age. (*CTP 87, 2037-39. Har 156.*)

5. (2) Depression in the elderly is common in conjunction with medical disabilities, especially cardiac problems, and is best supervised in a hospital. The use of tricyclics must be closely supervised because these medications cause excessive sedation, cardiac problems, and anticholinergic syndromes of the central or peripheral types such as urinary retention, narrow angle glaucoma, or confusion. A new antidepressive drug, bupropion (Wellbutrin), is unrelated to the tricyclics, and is associated with few cardiac problems but with increased seizure potential. (*CTP 1644-46, 1662. APA 1131-32. Har 671-72.*)

6. (5) Diabetes is the most common organic cause of a male erectile disorder. Primary organic impotence is uncommon, occurring in about 1% of men under age 35, whereas secondary (psychogenic) impotence is common and occurs in 10–20% of all men. Other organic etiologies include local disease of the genitals, vascular illness, neurological disease, endocrine disorders, systemic illness, and medications including over-the-counter and illegal drugs. (*CTP 1051. APA 596-97. Har 569.*)

7. (3) *Transsexualism* (gender dysphoria syndrome) is a disorder of gender identity. These individuals perceive themselves as being of the opposite sex. These subjects

are likely to cross-dress as children. They are not aroused erotically by wearing opposite-sex clothing. Three to four times more males than females apply for sex reassignment (surgical and medical treatment), but an equal number of males and females are actually reassigned.

There is a similar disorder called *transvestic fetishism* (a paraphilia), which usually involves a heterosexual male who has recurrent intense sexual urges and sexually arousing fantasies involving cross-dressing, often as an adjunct to masturbation or coitus. The disorder usually begins in childhood or early adolescence. The degree of assumed femininity usually is not as great as with transsexualism: when in male clothes, the transvestite male may appear hypermasculine. (*CTP 1075-76. APA 588-89.*)

8. **(1)** Family studies suggest a genetic predisposition in anorexia nervosa, with increased incidence of affective disorders in first-degree relatives. (See question 49 for details on anorexia.) (*CTP 1854-64. APA 755-59. Har 434-35.*)

9. **(3)** Hypothermia is a complication of anorexia in addition to other medical complications noted in question 56. (*CTP 1854-64. APA 756. Har 436.*)

10. **(1)** REM sleep is also called "Dreaming Sleep." In older adolescents and adults REM latency is shortened during major depressive episodes. REM changes noted over the lifespan are as follows: during the neonatal period, REM is 50% of total sleep and the infant goes from wakefulness directly to REM; at 4 months of age, REM drops to less than 40% of total sleep and starts after NREM; in young adulthood, REM is 25% of total sleep; in the elderly, there is some decrease in REM sleep.

L-tryptophan, a precursor of serotonin, hastens the onset of REM and NREM (seen in newborns from the high milk diet), whereas valine prolongs onset. Drugs that increase firing of norepinephrine-containing neurons cause a decrease in REM sleep. Dopamine has an alerting effect. Drugs increasing dopamine produce arousal and wakefulness, whereas dopamine blockers (pimozide, phenothiazines) increase sleep.

Brain acetylcholines (cholinergic-muscarinic agonists) increase REM sleep (seen in major depression), shorten REM latency (less than 60 minutes), and produce a greater percentage of REM with a shift of REM distribution from last half to first half of night. Reserpine produces depression and increases REM sleep. Antidepressants reduce REM sleep. Lack of sleep or restricted sleep improves depression.

Alzheimer's disease reduces REM and slow-wave sleep (stages 3 and 4). Narcolepsy and depression shorten REM latency. In mania, there is short sleep time in all phases and REM is greatly reduced. In schizophre-

nia, sleep is usually normal. Alcoholism and withdrawal from stimulants result in excessive sleep (hypersomnia). Insomnia is associated with tolerance to or withdrawal from CNS depressants.

Normal REM occurs after 90–100 minutes and reoccurs every 90–100 (some reference 60–100) minutes after NREM sleep (i.e., latency). Most time spent in REM is in the later one-third of night. REM periods increase after strong psychological stimuli (i.e., difficult learning, stress), and after use of chemicals and drugs that decrease brain catecholamines. (*CTP 1108-11. APA 743-49. Har 159-68.*)

11. **(5)** *Sleep apnea* refers to the apneic episode that occurs during sleep after the cessation of air flow at the nose or mouth lasting more than 10 seconds. Sleep apnea plays a role in crib deaths and deaths in adults, apparently as a result of arrhythmias and changes in blood pressure.

Adults with sleep apnea are likely to be middle-aged or older males who are tired and unable to stay awake in the daytime (42% have excessive somnolence). They may have an associated depression and mood changes. Physical findings in these patients include thick neck, weight gain (not necessarily obesity), increasing hypertension, and loud snoring at night. The history of sleep problems is usually obtained more specifically from the spouse or bed partner.

Obese patients with sleep apnea problems are said to have the Pickwickian syndrome (from the fat boy in Dickens' *Pickwick Papers*). (*CTP 1115. APA 764-67. Har 165-67.*)

12. **(3)** An individual's entire life is spent in three states: waking, NREM, and REM. Normal sleep patterns show sleep cycles every 70–100 minutes over 7 1/2 hours of sleep, with 4–6 NREM-REM cycles in each major sleep period. The elderly fall asleep earlier (an advance type of sleep schedule), whereas young adults have a delayed type of sleep schedule and fall asleep later. Slow-wave sleep (SWS) (stage 3 or 4) rebounds following sleep deprivation.

Advancing age (with reduction or loss of slow-wave sleep) decreases the ability to achieve long, uninterrupted periods of sleep or depth of sleep, resulting in an increased number of arousals. Daytime sleepiness occurs with increasing age (i.e., napping), along with increased nocturnal myoclonus, especially in older males. (See questions 10 and 61 for more details on sleep.) (*CTP 86-91. APA 740-42, 749. Har 152.*)

13. **(3)** Treatment of sleep apnea may involve medications to stimulate respiratory centers, mechanical tongue-retaining devices, and surgical procedures that can include tracheotomy and pharyngoplasty. The use of oxygen at night is of questionable value. Mechanical assistance for

respiration may be required. The patient must avoid antidepressant medication and alcohol.

Laboratory studies consist of polysomnographic recordings of 24 hours or all-night sleep, with EEG, EMG, and EKG monitoring and respiratory tracings to record air flow. (*CTP 1115. APA 746-47. Har 152-53.*)

14. (3) *Nocturnal myoclonus*, also called restless leg syndrome, is present when the subject is bothered by periodic movements during sleep, typically with sensations of creeping inside the calves whenever sitting or lying down, rarely painful, and the irresistible urge to move the legs. This condition interferes with sleep, resulting in insomnia and daytime tiredness. Sometimes it may be related to drugs (phenothiazines), pregnancy, and other medical problems. (*CTP 1116. APA 744-45. Har 166.*)

15. (4) *Sleep terrors*, "pavor nocturnus," "incubus," is a sleep arousal syndrome that typically occurs in the first third of the night during NREM (stages 3 and 4) and is manifested by a scream or cry and an intense anxiety reaction bordering on panic. The individual awakes in an disoriented state and does not remember the episode the next day. Sleep terrors are frequent in children and more common in males, and run in families. Sleep terrors do not indicate emotional illness. (*CTP 1121-22. Har 166.*)

16. (2) *Narcolepsy*, "sleep seizure," is a syndrome in which excessive daytime sleepiness results from abnormal frequent sleep-onset REM periods. There is a high familial incidence. It is most frequent in adolescents or young adults before age 30. There are four primary symptoms in narcolepsy:

1. an irresistible impulse for daytime naps or sleep attacks, where individuals cannot avoid falling asleep.
2. a sudden loss of muscle tension, *cataplexy*, with jaw drop, head drop, weakness of knees, and paralysis of all skeletal muscles with collapse. (About 75% of narcoleptics have cataplexy.)
3. sleep paralysis, where the individual is awake, conscious, but is unable to move muscles and may black out (become unconscious).
4. hypnagogic hallucinations.

Note: Cataplexy should not be confused with catalepsy, a generalized condition of diminished responsiveness usually characterized by a trance-like state, which can occur in organic, psychological disorders, or hypnosis. (*CTP 1116-17. APA 747-48. Har 123-24.*)

17. (5) *Acute intermittent porphyria*, the most common of the inherited porphyrias, is transmitted as an autosomal-dominant trait. Symptoms begin usually after puberty in the third or fourth decade of life. Women are more affected than men. Barbiturates, sulfonamides, griseofulvin, chloroquine, or certain steroids may precipitate attacks. Chronic symptoms frequently present are nervousness, anxiety, mood swings, emotional instability, angry outbursts, excitement, and psychotic behavior. Confusion, delirium, convulsions, and coma can develop during acute attacks. Common medical symptoms are abdominal crises, severe colic, paresthesias, and muscle weakness. (*CTP 1294.*)

18. (3) Pain is the most common complaint that brings patients to a physician. Underlying symptoms of chronic pain may be psychiatric problems such as depression, hypochondriasis, conversion disorder, compensation neurosis, malingering for secondary gain, and psychotic somatic delusions.

Treatment of chronic pain involves a multimodal approach by internists, surgeons, anesthesiologists, and psychiatrists. Placebos can decrease pain in one-third of individuals, so this effect does not necessarily differentiate between real and functional pain. Adequate analgesia is needed to treat pain: there is a tendency to underutilize narcotics, which should be given on a regular planned basis and not on a PRN basis in treating chronic pain. Psychotherapy, biofeedback, relaxation training, hypnosis, exercise, and nerve blocking have a place in the management of the patient with pain and may be part of a specialized chronic pain unit treatment program. (See question 23 reference placebos.) (*CTP 1268-69. APA 528-29. Har 412.*)

19. (3) *Postoperative delirium*, usually due to a combination of metabolic imbalances, anesthetic effects, and infections with or without fever, is particularly common in the elderly. Common causes include the stress of surgery, postoperative pain, insomnia, pain medication, electrolyte imbalance, infection, fever, and blood loss. Delirium is seen in about 10% of all hospital inpatients, 30% of patients in the surgical and coronary ICUs, and 20% of severely burned patients.

"*Black-patch*" delirium follows cataract surgery as a result of disorientation caused by covering the eyes. A small pinhole in the patch helps reduce or prevent the syndrome.

Dialysis dementia, a rare condition seen in patients who have been on dialysis for many years, presents with loss of memory, disorientation, dystonias, and seizures. The cause is unknown.

"*Sundowner*" syndrome manifests with drowsiness, confusion, ataxia, and falling. The syndrome, seen more often in the aged who are overly sedated and in the demented who are given small doses of psychoactive drugs, occurs when these patients experience reduced external stimuli when lights are reduced at night or when they are socially isolated.

Pseudodementia occurs in the depressed elderly who manifest memory impairment or other cognitive defects that disappear with the treatment of the depression. (*CTP 1196. Har 363.*)

20. (1) Chronic hemodialysis can result in problems of dependency on others, depression, suicide, and sexual problems that can be both neurogenic and psychogenic. (See question 19 regarding dialysis dementia.) (*CTP 1318.*)

21. (5) Laboratory values in hypothyroidism reveal a low serum T_3 and T_4 but an elevated TSH. Hypothyroidism is usually of an insidious onset. The patient feels slowed down and lethargic with many signs and symptoms of depression. About 10% of these patients can develop a full-blown psychotic disorder called "myxedema madness." Before overt symptoms of hypothyroidism are seen, a patient with Grade III, subclinical Hashimoto thyroiditis (with antithyroid antibodies) may have psychiatric symptoms including depression, paranoia, irritability, and confusion. Hypothyroidism can mimic psychotic depression, paranoid schizophrenia, and manic depression. (*CTP 1213. APA 525. Har 135, 373.*)

22. (4) Delirium, characterized by the patient's inability to attend, is manifested by fluctuations in the level of arousal, orientation, attention, perceptions, and affect. Delirium is most often acute and severe, but can be subacute and mild, especially when caused by a chronic fungal encephalomeningitis or by the toxic effects of many psychotropic medications. (See question 75 reference delirium and dementia.) (*CTP 624-29. APA 282-84. Har 361-62.*)

23. (2) Naloxone can block the analgesic effect of a placebo, suggesting that the release of endogenous opioids may explain some placebo effects. The use of placebos can be considered deceptive treatment and may seriously undermine the patient's confidence in the physician. The use of placebos can lead to dependence on pill-taking and can result in various adverse side effects. (See question 18.) (*CTP 1289-90. APA 528.*)

24. (3) Multiple sclerosis causes diffuse multifocal lesions in the white matter of the CNS. It occurs more frequently in the cold and temperate climates, and in women and young adults (20-40 years). Symptoms consist of weakness, ataxia, diffuse sensory and motor abnormalities, and vision changes. Mental disturbances are present in about 50% of patients. Various CNS changes can suggest a psychiatric disorder such as a hysteria or a conversion reaction. (*CTP 191-92, 1295.*)

25. (3) *Hyperventilation syndrome* is produced by increased respirations beyond the respiratory frequency and depth needed to maintain blood gases in the normal range, with resulting blowing off of CO_2. The decreased CO_2 in blood circulation produces a respiratory alkalosis causing bicarbonate to move out of plasma; calcium then becomes less ionized resulting in neuromuscular symptoms. In addition, there is reduced cerebral blood flow,

due to the respiratory alkalosis, causing a slow, high-voltage EEG.

Hyperventilation syndrome is relatively common and is typically due to anxiety. Focal neurological symptoms, carpopedal spasms, and tetany may mimic other disorders. Deliberate hyperventilation will reproduce the symptoms. Treatment consists of having the patient breathe into a plastic or paper bag to reduce the CO_2 depletion, and this relieves the symptoms. (*CTP 1198-99. APA 502.*)

26. (2) Normal grieving and pathological depression share many common features. Grief-stricken patients who are physically ill do not have unreasonable grief, do not generalize their medical problems, do not have a sense of personal worthlessness, and do not lack confidence in facing the future. On the other hand, depressed patients with a physical illness have lower self-esteem, and feel frustrated, helpless, or guilty. (*CTP 1346. APA 300. Har 747-49.*)

27. (4) Kubler-Ross (1969) presented five stages of dying. The stages are not unique to dying and are seen in other losses. Fear and anxiety are not represented in the stages.
    Stage 1. Shock and denial—Some do not go beyond this stage and are difficult to manage.
    Stage 2. Anger—"Why me," angry at God, or fate.
    Stage 3. Bargaining—May give to charity.
    Stage 4. Depression—Shows clinical signs.
    Stage 5. Acceptance—Realizes death is inevitable.
    (*CTP 1340-41. Har 729-31.*)

28. (C) Psychological tests, such as the Wechsler Adult Intelligence Scale (WAIS), in the elderly, show that verbal performance is maintained with age, but perceptual motor skills decline. With the elderly, cognitive problems (memory, perception, thinking) are more likely. Learning new material takes longer, but there is no significant decrease in intelligence. (*CTP 2022-24. Har 667.*)

29. (E) In aging there is increased incidence of atrophic gastritis, hiatal hernias, and diverticulosis, with wrinkling of the skin, loss of subcutaneous fat, decrease in melanin, and loss of sweat glands. Visual changes are common with a decrease in acuity, peripheral vision, and night vision. The aged show more refractory errors and an increased prevalence of cataracts and glaucoma. (*CTP 2037-40. Har 666-67.*)

30. (E) AIDS (acquired immune deficiency syndrome) is a significant cause of dementia and intellectual deterioration, and predisposes to intracranial infections and neoplasms. (*CTP 1297-1316. Har 371. APA 290.*)

31. (D) HIV-III (human immunodeficiency virus) is infectious and is directly transmitted through blood contain-

ing body fluids and semen. (*CTP 1297-1316. Har 371. APA 290.*)

32. **(E)** There is a direct HIV-III infection of the nervous system causing various CNS changes. (See question 30.) (*CTP 1308. APA 290. Har 371.*)

33. **(B)** Antianxiety medications in the elderly are relatively free of dangerous side effects when used in low dosage for short periods of time.

The longer acting anxiolytics are more likely to cause problems with the elderly. Older patients are prone to drug accumulation with unwanted sedative or central inhibitory effects, which can cause intellectual changes. Clearance of the benzodiazepines is delayed in the elderly because of the high lipid solubility of these medications and the age-related increase in the proportion of adipose tissue. Delayed hepatic metabolism also plays a role in drug accumulation. As a result, motor incoordination and delirium can occur as increasing accumulation builds up to toxic levels of the drugs.

Barbiturates are to be avoided with older patients as these medications suppress REM sleep. Chloral hydrate can aggravate gastric ulceration. Propranolol may add to sleep problems as insomnia and vivid dreams are potential side effects. (*CTP 2040-41. APA 1135-36. Har 677-78.*)

34. **(E)** Confusion in the elderly can be caused by various drugs such as transdermal scopolamine, eye drops containing atropine, cimetidine, ibuprofen, indomethacin, levodopa, timolol, trazodone, and rantidine (Zantac). (*CTP 2050. Har 672.*)

35. **(B)** *Dementia* manifests with deterioration of memory, general intellectual and specific cognitive capacities, and social functioning. Dementia arises after normal intellectual maturity has been reached. Despite these mental changes in dementia, consciousness remains full and clear. (*APA 1118. CTP 612-24. Har 366-67.*)

36. **(A)** *Multi-infarct dementia*, compared with Alzheimer's disease, has a sudden, stepwise pattern of increasing disability with islands of preserved function. In multi-infarct dementia, neurological motor signs and asymmetries, hypertension, a history or evidence of stroke, arteriosclerotic damage at other sites, and accompanying depression are likely to be present. It occurs in about 15% of dementia cases in the elderly and is more frequent in men than in women. (*CTP 617-20. APA 1119. Har 369.*)

37. **(E)** Depression, in contrast to dementia, is likely to have a more acute onset of cognitive symptoms and less correlation with physical disability, age, or duration of illness. The depressed patients show concern, are well-oriented, but do not try hard to succeed at tests of memory,

unless coached into answering; their complaints exceed the objective signs of deficits. Demented patients, by contrast, may confabulate and are unable to answer tests of memory, even with much encouragement. Dementia occurs mostly in old age, and in relation to organic causes. (*CTP 621-22. APA 1129-30. Har 376-77.*)

38. **(B)** The elderly have reduced renal clearance, which can result in increased lithium blood levels. (See questions 33 and 39.) (*CTP 2037-45. APA 1117-39. Har 677-78.*)

39. **(A)** The use of lithium in the elderly needs to be monitored closely, keeping the target dose at the low end of usually therapeutic blood levels. Doses larger than 900 mg per day generally are not required as renal filtration drops progressively with age. Thiazide diuretics and salt and water restriction are likely to produce increased lithium blood levels. (*CTP 2044-45. APA 1132-33. Har 675.*)

40. **(A)** The same dose ranges of antidepressants can be used in the elderly as with other ages, but overall levels should be on the low side. The starting doses should be half or less of the adult standard and further doses slowly increased. The side effects must be monitored more closely as any minor ones, such as dry mouth, constipation, blurred vision, tremor, and unsteadiness, may increase the likelihood of noncompliance. The elderly are more prone to constipation, urinary problems, and cardiac conduction deficits. (*CTP 1638, 2042-44. APA 1131-33. Har 676.*)

41. **(B)** *Sexual dysfunction disorders* occur at a prevalence in all adults of 35–40%, with male erectile problems of 10–20%, hypoactive sexual desire in both male and females of 1–35%, inhibited orgasm in 5–30% females and 5% males. At some point in life, 50% of men and 77% of women report sexual difficulties including a lack of interest or an inability to relax during sexual activity.

The true incidence of premature ejaculation has not been determined. Twenty to thirty percent of all men at some time encounter the problem. It is more common among college educated men than among those less educated. A stressful marriage is likely to exacerbate the disorder. Treatment of premature ejaculation is usually by practice of the squeeze technique or the stop-start technique (Semans, 1956). (*CTP 1054. APA 599-600. Har 573.*)

42. **(A)** Amenorrhea can occur in a physically healthy adult and is referred to as idiopathic amenorrhea. Amenorrhea may be a manifestation of psychiatric syndromes such as anorexia nervosa and pseudocyesis, other physical conditions such as obesity, diseases of the pituitary and hypothalamus, or secondary to excessive running and jogging, certain drugs (reserpine, chlorpromazine), and following a course of ECT. (*APA 785-86.*)

43. **(A)** About every 90 minutes during REM, men experience penile erection, nocturnal penile tumescence, which can be documented by a strain gauge. Other assessment procedures include doppler flow studies, penile blood pressure measurements, arteriography and papaverine injections of the corpora cavernosa to assess for vascular competence, and nerve root stimulation to assess for neurological impairments. Many drugs can impair erection and ejaculation, including psychiatric medications, antihypertensives, and commonly abused drugs. Although many physical diseases also can injure the erection mechanism, some reports claim that 90% of all cases of impotence are of a psychological nature. (*CTP 1051. APA 597. Har 569-70.*)

44. **(E)** Impotence can be caused by psychological factors, such as conflictual feelings of desire, a punitive superego, an inability to trust, feelings of inadequacy, or a sense of being undesirable. Fear, performance anxiety, anger, or moral prohibition may also be factors.

    Other causes of impotence to consider are homosexual orientation or history of incest, sexual trauma, sexual abuse, or rape. Psychiatric diseases such as depression and schizophrenia, and medical conditions, especially vascular insufficiency, metabolic problems, liver and kidney diseases, all play a factor in impotence. In the elderly, the lack of a sexual partner is a common factor. (See questions 6 and 43.) (*CTP 1051-52. APA 596-97. Har 569.*)

45. **(E)** Drugs that affect erectile functions:

    Abused drugs—alcohol, opiates, cocaine
    Antihypertensives—clonidine, propranolol, methyldopa, hydrochlorthiazide
    Antidepressants—trazodone can give priaprism
    Antipsychotics—fluphenazine, thioridazine, reserpine
    Other drugs—lithium, amphetamines, steroids, estrogens, cimetidine, antiparkinsonian agents (See question 43.) (*CTP 1052. APA 595-99. Har 569-70.*)

46. **(B)** *Pedophilia*, the recurrent intense sexual urge directed toward or aroused by young children, is a major subcategory of paraphilias. Fifty percent of the pedophiles develop paraphilic arousal prior to age 18. Ninety percent of the offenders are male. The vast majority of acts against victims involve genital fondling or oral sex. Vaginal or anal penetration is infrequent except in cases of incest. A significant number of pedophiles are involved in exhibitionism, voyeurism, or rape.

    There is no specific treatment. These subjects have been treated with antiandrogenic medications, antipsychotics, antiaggressive medications (lithium, Tegretol, clonazepine), and chemical castration (Depo-Provera). However, one-third of castrated men can still engage in sexual activity including intercourse. (*CTP 1076-77. APA 592-95. Har 84.*)

47. **(E)** The legal definition of rape is penetration (even slight) in sexual intercourse against the victim's will and consent. Sodomy is defined as fellatio and anal penetration. Rape is usually an act of violence and humiliation, an expression of power or anger, expressed through sexual means.

    Rape is a highly unreported crime as only one in four to one in ten are reported. After a rape, the female victim generally feels shame, humiliation, confusion, fear, and rage, and many develop post-traumatic stress disorder. Male rape is defined as sodomy. Homosexual rape is more frequent with men than females, and usually occurs in closed institutions such as prisons and maximum security hospitals. Men who are sexually attacked feel similar to women who have been raped, and many fear they will become homosexuals. (*CTP 1096-99.*)

48. **(A)** See question 46. (*CTP 1081. APA 592-95.*)

49. **(B)** Anorexia nervosa patients generally lose weight by decreasing food intake, through taking decreased portions of high carbohydrate and fat-containing foods. Others use some form of a rigorous exercise program, self-induced vomiting, laxative and diuretic abuse, and other purging behaviors to lose or keep weight down.

    The treatment goal is to restore the patient's nutritional state to normal. Treatment modalities include behavioral and operant conditioning based on weight gain using as positive reinforcers increased activity, visiting privileges, and social activities. Medications, and cognitive and family therapy must also be considered. (*CTP 1862-63. APA 758-59. Har 436.*)

50. **(B)** There are two types of eating disorders resulting in weight loss—bingeing and purging, and restricting food intake by fasting. Bulimic anorectics are less regressed in sexual activity than anorectics, and may be promiscuous. They are more likely to have personality disorders manifested by impulsive behavior, such as suicide attempts, self-mutilation, stealing, and substance abuse. (*APA 756. Har 435.*)

51. **(E)** Obesity is not considered a psychiatric diagnosis, as there is no distinct psychopathology of obesity. It is related to socioeconomic status and is more common with females of low economic status and increasing age up to age 50. If both parents are obese, 80% of children become obese, with one obese parent 40% of children are obese, and only 10% become obese with lean parents. Obese individuals have a greater number of fat cells. (*CTP 1179-86. APA 763-66.*)

52. **(E)** In the treatment of mild obesity, 20–40% overweight, the most efficient methods are behavior modification in a group setting, a balanced diet, and exercise. With moderate obesity, 41–100% overweight, individually supervised protein-sparing modified fasting with 400–700 calories a day is

needed. Behavior treatment that includes self-monitoring, nutrition education, physical activity, and cognitive restructuring may be of value. Medications may be helpful (fenfuramine, phenylpropanolamine), but there can be a rebound effect. Severe or morbid obesity, greater than 100% over normal weight, is the least common form of obesity: treatment may be in the form of surgery to decrease the size of stomach or produce a bypass.

With children, behavior modification may be used and must involve the school and parents. Psychotherapy is generally not very effective. (*CTP 1178-86. APA 764-65. Har 536.*)

53. **(B)** After gastrointestinal bypass surgery, complications may occur in both personal and interpersonal relationships, but often the patient does much better than using diet alone. (See question 52.) (*APA 765. CTP 1184-85. Har 536.*)

54. **(E)** See question 50. (*CTP 1854-64. APA 760-63. Har 435.*)

55. **(E)** With bulimia, vomiting or the use of diuretics and laxatives can cause hypokalemia alkalosis and metabolic acidosis. Fasting results in dehydration, increased potassium excretion, weakness, lethargy, and, at times, cardiac arrhythmias which can lead to cardiac arrest (also from vomiting and diuretics complications).

Cardiac failure due to a cardiomyopathy from ipecac (emetine) intoxication is a serious consequence. Other problems that may be seen are severe attrition and erosion of the teeth, parotid gland enlargement, acute dilation of stomach (rare emergency), and esophageal tears. (*CTP 1860. APA 760-63.*)

56. **(A)** Medical complications are secondary to starvation or purging (self-induced vomiting, laxative, and diuretic abuse, other purging). Other complications that can occur are leukopenia with relative lymphocytosis, hypokalemic alkalosis leading to weakness and lethargy, and at times, cardiac arrhythmias and cardiac arrest. Amenorrhea may be seen before weight loss. Poor sexual adjustment is common. (See question 49.) (*CTP 1854-64. APA 755-59. Har 436.*)

57. **(D)** Excessive caffeine use can result in sleep problems. If used before sleep, caffeine decreases total slow-wave sleep. CNS stimulants and other medications used for weight reduction cause insomnia, as do antimetabolites, thyroid preparations, anticonvulsants, monoamine oxidase inhibitors, ACTH, oral contraceptives, and beta-blocking drugs.

Insomnia occurs after and during withdrawal from drugs with sedative or tranquilizing properties such as benzodiazepines, phenothiazines, sedating tricyclics, illegal drugs (marijuana), opiates, alcohol, and CNS depressants. (*CTP 1110. Har 164.*)

58. **(B)** See questions 11 and 59 referring to sleep apnea. (*CTP 1115. APA 746-47. Har 165-67.*)

59. **(E)** Problems with *sleep apnea* include tiredness, poor job performance, mood changes, auto accidents, impotence, and decreased libido. (See question 3.) (*CTP 1115. APA 746-47. Har 165-67.*)

60. **(D)** Treatment of insomnia includes proper sleep hygiene with a regular sleep schedule, light exercise daily, control of sounds and hunger, and the avoidance of caffeinated beverages, alcohol, and tobacco in the evenings. (*CTP 1108. APA 742. Har 165.*)

61. **(E)** Worriers sleep more and are classified as "long sleepers" (more than nine hours a day), whereas "short sleepers" (less than six hours a day) are generally normal, rested, and satisfied with life. Sleep needs vary little across cultures and geographic areas and are usually seven and a half hours daily (six hours in NREM, one and a half hours in REM). Humans are normally unable to reduce the amount of sleep to under five to six hours per day. (*CTP 91-92, 1106-11. APA 741-52. Har 156, 158-60.*)

62. **(C)** Manic and depressed individuals have unusual sleep patterns. The manic phase has a short sleep time, especially in REM, but stage 4 is about normal. (See question 64.) During depression, there is insomnia, difficulty in remaining asleep rather than in falling asleep. In addition, there are frequent awakenings at night and early morning, reduced slow-wave sleep and REM latency, and an increased requirement for sleep and REM sleep. (*CTP 1109-10. APA 748. Har 160-61.*)

63. **(A)** Polysomnographic examination is used to study sleep patterns. A sleep laboratory evaluation is usually not indicated in the diagnosis of the most common parasomnias but may be helpful in nocturnal epilepsy, nocturnal panic attacks, sleep-disordered breathing, epileptogenic parasomnia, myoclonic sleep disorders, narcolepsy, or sleep apnea. (*CTP 1105-18. APA 750. Har 153.*)

64. **(A)** Manic patients have difficulty falling asleep but do not complain of sleep problems. They feel refreshed after two to four hours of sleep and have a decreased need for sleep. (See question 62.) (*CTP 906, 1109. Har 160-61.*)

65. **(E)** Family incidence is increased in patients with parasomnias of childhood, especially sleepwalking, sleep terrors, functional enuresis (nocturnal type), bruxism (tooth grinding), and myoclonus syndrome. (*CTP 1116. APA 749-50.*)

66. **(B)** The diagnosis of myoclonic sleep disorder is made by polygraph recordings with surface electrodes placed

primarily over the tibialis muscles along with other muscle groups. (See question 14.) (*CTP 1111, 1116. APA 744-45. Har 166.*)

67. **(B)** Normal sleep with aging, see question 12. (*CTP 87. APA 740-41. Har 152.*)

68. **(B)** The treatment of narcolepsy is by the use of psychostimulants, such as amphetamine or methylphenidate, and sometimes with antidepressants (such as protriptyline—Vivactil).

    The Kleine-Levin syndrome, which is rare and is seen in male adolescents, must be considered in the differential diagnosis. The syndrome consists of three to four episodes per year of hypersomnia, hyperactivity, bulimia, increased masturbation, outbursts of belligerence, and sometimes hallucinations. (See question 16.) (*CTP 558, 1116-17. APA 747-48. Har 124.*)

69. **(C)** Chronic alcoholism results in excessive sleep (hypersomnia) during night and daytime, even after stopping drinking. There is a loss of slow-wave sleep and impaired sleep continuity. Other disorders that show similar patterns are anxiety disorders, affective disorders, schizophrenia, and drug abuse. (*CTP 1111. APA 749. Har 163-65.*)

70. **(C)** The management of chronic pain is discussed in question 18. (*CTP 1189-90, 1268-71. APA 528-29. Har 412.*)

71. **(E)** *Myocardial infarction* has been reported to be associated with a "Type A" behavior pattern, elevated cholesterol levels, cigarette smoking, and hypertension. During recovery, there is usually initial denial; then anxiety alternating with denial occurs after a few days; usually next, the patient realizes that he or she will probably survive, and depression develops. Denial improves the prognosis. Near the time of discharge or shortly thereafter, a homecoming depression frequently occurs.

    Antianxiety drugs (diazepine or propranolol) are of value in the acute postinfarction period to prevent arrhythmias from excessive anxiety due to increased catecholamines.

    Antidepressants or stimulants are medically dangerous in the postinfarction period, but can be considered after six to eight weeks. Exercise and coitus can begin in a progressive manner after discharge from hospital. (*CTP 1194-96. APA 499-501. Har 237-38.*)

72. **(A)** In patients with obstructive pulmonary disease, increased emotional problems (anxiety and depression) worsen the dypsnea and the hypoxia, thus decreasing cognitive efficiency. (*CTP 1207-9.*)

73. **(B)** Although symptoms of depression and dementia generally occur in Parkinson's disease (dementia seen in 30–80% of cases) and Huntington's chorea, intellectual deterioration usually precedes depression. The most common neurological syndromes manifesting depressive symptoms are Parkinson's disease (50–70% of patients), Alzheimer's disease, epilepsy, strokes, and tumors. (*CTP 208, 632. APA 1119. Har 375.*)

74. **(A)** In systemic lupus erythematosus, drugs such as d-methyldopa and chlorpromazine may produce mental confusion in a few cases; however, 15–50% of patients with this illness have abnormal mental functions ranging from acute psychosis with disorientation, confusion, inattention, delusions, and hallucinations to chronic progressive dementia. (*CTP 633-34, 1295. APA 507.*)

75. **(A)** Dementia, when compared with delirium, has less hour-to-hour fluctuation in cognitive functions. The difference is more quantitative than qualitative as the two conditions can coexist. The cardinal feature of delirium is day-to-day, hour-to-hour, and minute-to-minute fluctuation in brain dysfunction. (*CTP 627-28. APA 283-84. Har 361-62.*)

76. **(E)** Delirium is characterized by a sudden onset of symptoms with a disturbance of the sleep-wake cycle, a reduced level of consciousness, and a change of motor activity along with memory and orientation problems. Haloperidol in low doses is the drug of choice for agitated, restless, fearful, or belligerent behavior. Short-acting benzodiazepines such as triazolam (Halcion) are helpful for insomnia. (See question 19.) (*CTP 626-27. Har 363.*)

77. **(D)** Patients with delirium may become more confused when placed in the strange setting of an intensive care unit or during the evening when cues are diminished (sundowning). About one-quarter of hospitalized patients with delirium die within three or four months. (See question 76.) (*CTP 628-29. APA 283.*)

78. **(E)** Delirium can occur in patients treated with psychotropics (anticholinergic delirium) and other medications such as the anti-ulcer agent cimetidine. It occurs most frequently in the aged and children, and in those with preexisting brain damage or a history of delirium. (*CTP 625-26. Har 362-63.*)

79. **(E)** *Organic mood disorder* (previously called organic affective syndrome) has a insidious onset, history of depression, accentuation by psychosocial stressors, and an absence of cognitive impairment. The causes include endocrinopathies (hypothyroidism, Cushing's syndrome, Addison's disease, hyperparathyroidism), infectious diseases, systemic diseases such as renal or hepatic failure, pernicious anemia, systemic lupus erythematosis, parkinsonism, chronic obstructive pulmonary disease, viral infections, and malignancies. Neurological disease

as a cause can either be intracranial or extracranial. Many drugs such as reserpine, corticosteroids, methyldopa, oral contraceptives, amphetamines, hallucinogens, and over-the-counter and illicit drugs are also etiological factors. (*CTP 630-33. APA 290. Har 381.*)

80. **(D)** Sterilization, vasectomy, salpingectomy and ligation of the fallopian tubes have a low morbidity and mortality. A small proportion of patients may suffer a neurotic poststerilization syndrome, manifested by hypochondriasis, pain, loss of libido, sexual unresponsiveness, depression, and concerns over masculinity or femininity. After a hysterectomy, there can be a fear of loss of sexual attractiveness with sexual dysfunction in a small percentage of women.

    Prostatectomy commonly results in sexual dysfunction and, depending on the surgical procedure used, may lead to absence of emission, ejaculation, and erection. The patient may need a penile implant. About one-third of patients after a colostomy feel worse about themselves and manifest shame and self-consciousness. Phantom limb phenomenon occurs in 98% of cases after surgical amputation or removal. (*CTP 1328.*)

81. **(A)** Hyperventilation can be seen in multiple sclerosis, cerebrovascular accidents, myocardial infarction, transient cardiac ischemic events and arrhythmias, epilepsy, hypoglycemia, hysteria, vasovagal or hypoglycemic attacks, bronchial asthma, acute porphyria, Meniere's disease, and pheochromocytoma. The psychiatric causes include anxiety attacks, panic attacks, schizophrenia, borderline or histrionic personality disorders, and phobic or obsessive disorders. (See question 25.) (*CTP 1198-99. APA 503.*)

82. **(C)** After a myocardial infarction, there is usually anxiety, denial, and depression. (See question 71.) (*CTP 1194-95. APA 500. Har 237–38.*)

83. **(A)** Hospital discharge after recovering from a myocardial infarction is likely to precipitate increased psychological distress, the so-called "homecoming depression." The prognosis is better if postinfarction denial has allowed less overt anxiety. Tricyclic antidepressants are usually safe to use after six to eight weeks postinfarction if there are no serious cardiac conduction problems. (See question 71.) (*CTP 1193-96. APA 497-501. Har 237-38.*)

5

PSYCHOTHERAPY

1. All of the following are characteristic of Malan's brief psychotherapy except:

    1. Limited number of sessions
    2. Agreed treatment focus
    3. Less attention to transference
    4. Strong patient motivation for change
    5. Patient able to think in psychological terms

2. Which of the following statements regarding the outcome of different psychotherapies is correct?

    1. No one type of psychotherapy is most effective
    2. The majority of psychotherapies have no long-term beneficial effects
    3. Patients randomly assigned to control and psychotherapy treatment groups showed no difference in results
    4. Medication tends to nullify the effect of psychotherapy
    5. Cognitive behavioral psychotherapy is more effective than antidepressant in relieving depression.

3. Which of the following techniques is least likely to be used in psychoanalysis?

    1. Free association
    2. Analyst neutrality
    3. Confrontation
    4. Therapeutic guidance
    5. Interpretation

4. Which of the following syndromes would be least likely to respond favorably to psychoanalysis?

    1. Dysthymic disorder
    2. Paranoid personality disorder
    3. Phobic disorder
    4. Obsessive compulsive disorder
    5. Generalized anxiety disorder

5. All of the following statements about primary process thinking are correct except:

    1. Characteristically occurs in dreams
    2. Not bound by time sequence
    3. In wake state, should not occur in emotionally stable adult

    4. Primarily nonverbal
    5. Concerned with wish-fulfillment

6. In cognitive therapy, all of the following techniques are used except:

    1. Rehearsing behaviors
    2. Assigning homework
    3. Identifying automatic thoughts
    4. Encouraging ventilation of feelings
    5. Correcting cognitive distortions

7. All of the following statements about hypnosis are correct except:

    1. Severely depressed patients are not readily hypnotized
    2. Self-hypnosis is an effective treatment for recurrent phobia
    3. Electroencephalogram shows delta waves during hypnotic trance
    4. Preanesthetic hypnosis results in lowered level of anesthesia required
    5. Hypnosis is used to recover memory loss in psychogenic amnesia

8. A physician refuses to work with alcoholic patients. He states that they are manipulative, unmotivated for change, and overly dependent. The doctor's attitude is an example of:

    1. Projective identification
    2. Intellectualization
    3. Reaction formation
    4. Counterphobia
    5. Countertransference

DIRECTIONS: For questions 9 through 35, one or more of the alternatives given are correct. After you decide which alternatives are correct, record your selection according to the following key.

(A) if alternatives 1, 2 and 3 only are correct.
(B) if alternatives 1 and 3 only are correct.
(C) if alternatives 2 and 4 only are correct.
(D) if alternative 4 only is correct.
(E) if all four alternatives are correct.

9. According to behavior therapy principles, which of the following are correct?

1. Reinforcement that occurs only occasionally will maintain target behavior
2. Underlying emotions must be dealt with before behavior change will occur
3. Maladaptive behavior is learned by same methods as adaptive behavior
4. The expectations of a subject have little effect on the outcome

10. In treating agoraphobia with behavior therapy, which of the following statements are correct?

    1. Direct, in vivo exposure is more effective than exposure in imagination
    2. Flooding is more effective in reducing symptoms quickly
    3. Patients can efficiently self-regulate their exposure by computer
    4. Many patients develop alternative substitute symptoms

11. A learned response is more likely to be extinguished when:

    1. Reinforcement is only occasional
    2. Paired with reciprocal, contrasting response
    3. Exposure to feared stimulus is delayed until the patient is relaxed
    4. Patient is motivated for change

12. Cognitive therapy would be appropriate treatment for patients with:

    1. Borderline personality disorder
    2. Primary degenerative dementia
    3. Residual schizophrenia
    4. Depression following myocardial infarction

13. According to the cognitive model for depression, which of the following are considered factors underlying depression?

    1. Negative self-image
    2. Anger introjected
    3. Pessimistic anticipation
    4. Early deprivation

14. Which of the following statements regarding family therapy are correct?

    1. Therapy can proceed without all family members present
    2. Involves treatment across generations
    3. More effective than group therapy with phobic patients
    4. Contraindicated with psychotic patients

15. In behavioral therapy, which of the following are important procedures?

1. Defining specific problems requiring therapy
2. Clarifying underlying unconscious causes
3. Understanding environmental factors maintaining the problem
4. Interpreting dynamic process

16. Which of the following statements about group therapy with schizophrenics are correct?

    1. As measured by readmission rates, individual therapy is more effective than group therapy
    2. Supportive groups are more beneficial than interpretive groups
    3. Most effective during inpatient phase of treatment
    4. Tends to be more leader oriented than peer oriented

17. Which of the following techniques are used in structural family therapy (Minuchin)?

    1. Enacting rather than describing family behavior
    2. Problem is paradoxically redefined as being useful
    3. Organizing the family into subgroups
    4. Assignment of roles and tasks outside of sessions

18. The advantages of having cotherapists in group therapy includes which of the following?

    1. Simulates parents of family
    2. Presents different theoretical approaches
    3. Minimizes countertransference blind spots
    4. Decreases patients' unrealistic transference

19. During supportive psychotherapy, which of the following occur?

    1. Resolution of pregenital conflicts
    2. Working through of transference
    3. Therapeutic regression fostered
    4. Strengthening existing ego state

20. Which of the following are characteristic of the termination phase of psychoanalysis?

    1. Involves analysis of the transference
    2. Patient mourns impending loss of analyst
    3. Working through of countertransference
    4. Separation anxiety often occurs

21. In supportive psychotherapy, which of the following techniques are used?

    1. Support
    2. Education
    3. Encouragement
    4. Neutrality

22. When brief dynamic psychotherapy is compared with long-term psychoanalytic psychotherapy, which of the following statements are correct?

    1. Transference is ignored in brief therapy
    2. Therapist is nonjudgmental in both

3. Confrontation used only in long-term psychotherapy
4. A focal problem is selected in brief therapy

23. Appropriate goals of group therapy are likely to include which of the following?

    1. Support
    2. Reality testing
    3. Vicarious learning
    4. Control of violent behavior

24. Which of the following statements are correct in the management of patients with narcissistic personality disorder?

    1. Tend to both idealize and depreciate the therapist
    2. Symptoms similar to antisocial personality disorder
    3. React intensely to criticism
    4. Psychodynamic psychotherapy is contraindicated

25. Which of the following techniques are appropriate in group therapy?

    1. Interpretation
    2. Videotape playback
    3. Free association
    4. Confrontation

26. Which of the following patient syndromes are most often treated in heterogeneous therapy groups?

    1. Schizoid personality
    2. Post-traumatic stress disorder
    3. Somatoform disorder
    4. Antisocial personality disorder

27. In psychoanalysis, which of the following statements regarding working through are correct?

    1. Involves exploration of interpretation
    2. Insight is confirmed against external reality
    3. Material is integrated with patient's ego
    4. When present, indicates analysis is in termination phase

28. To facilitate a therapeutic alliance, the analyst should:

    1. Avoid confrontation
    2. Avoid early discussion of fees
    3. Offer early reassurance
    4. Provide a confidential process

29. During an analysis, which of the following are likely to indicate countertransference in the analyst?

    1. Repeated drowsiness during sessions
    2. Allowing the patient to stay longer than scheduled time
    3. Forgetting the patient's name
    4. Terminating the session when patient threatens physical violence

30. Which of the following statements about countertransference are correct?

    1. May be used by the analyst to gain insight into the patient's interactions
    2. Inevitably present during course of analysis
    3. Removes analyst's necessary neutrality
    4. May necessitate analyst returning to own analysis

31. Which of the following are prerequisites for a patient about to undertake psychoanalysis?

    1. Strong motivation
    2. Ability for self-observation
    3. Ability to form relationships
    4. Good ego strength

32. In the process of a productive psychoanalysis, which of the following occur?

    1. Transference neurosis
    2. Working through
    3. Dream interpretation
    4. Analysis of the countertransference

33. In psychodynamic psychotherapies, which of the following abilities are necessary for the patient's participation?

    1. Ability to regress
    2. Ability to form a therapeutic alliance
    3. Ability to benefit without medication
    4. Ability to utilize insight

34. Which of the following statements regarding free association are correct in psychoanalysis?

    1. May be blocked by development of transference
    2. Promoted by lying on the couch
    3. Liable to be blocked by resistance
    4. Facilitated by correct interpretation

35. Which of the following statements about interpersonal psychotherapy for depression are correct?

    1. Antidepressant medication relieves the same symptoms
    2. Focuses on symptom relief rather than personality change
    3. Therapist neutral to maximize transference
    4. Typically weekly sessions limited to three to four months' total duration

ANSWERS AND EXPLANATIONS

1. (3) David Malan and the Tavistock Group described the goals of brief psychotherapy as: (1) clarify the nature of the defense, the anxiety, and the impulse, and (2) link the present, past, and transference.

   The patient must be highly motivated, be able to "think in feeling terms," and have a good response to trial interpretations. The therapeutic focus is on the internal conflicts present since childhood. A termination date must be set up at the beginning of treatment. (See question 22 for more details on brief psychotherapy.) (*CTP 1564-67. APA 861-62. Har 591.*)

2. (1) Psychotherapy is a general term for a large number of treatment techniques in which the primary means of effecting perceptual and behavior changes is through verbal interchange and the reorganization of mental structures.

   The effectiveness of psychotherapy is still a subject of debate. It is still unclear how to decide which psychotherapy is suitable for which patient and by which therapist. (*CTP 1570-73. APA 855-56. Har 450.*)

3. (3) Psychoanalytic techniques consist of free association, therapeutic alliance, neutrality, abstinence, defense analysis, and the interpretation of transference. (See question 20 for more details.) (*CTP 1452-57. APA 858. Har 459.*)

4. (2) Psychoanalysis can be useful in the treatment of obsessional and anxiety disorders, dysthymia, moderately severe personality disorders, impulse disorders, paraphilias, and other sexual disorders. (*CTP 1454-55. APA 857-59. Har 459.*)

5. (3) Primary process thinking (irrational system) is motivated by the pleasure principle (Freud), where an idea and its opposite may coexist. The mental contents are condensed, displaced freely and concerned with wishfulfillment. Primary process thinking occurs in dreams and psychosis, and is primarily nonverbal.

   Secondary process (rational) thinking is based on the reality principle. (*CTP 369, 560. APA 126-27. Har 173.*)

6. (4) Cognitive therapy techniques, sometimes referred to as "collaborative empiricism," consist of structured and directive tasks such as assigned readings and homework, along with behavioral techniques including identification of irrational beliefs, attitudes, automatic thoughts, and assumptions that underlie negatively biased thoughts. (See questions 12 and 13 for more details on cognitive therapy.) (*CTP 1541-50. APA 869-72. Har 536-40.*)

7. (3) There is no known biological basis for hypnosis as measured in EEG and physiological changes of sleep. The essential feature of hypnosis is the subjective experiential changes that occur. Self-hypnosis (autogenic training) can be taught to help a patient relax. Hypnosis can be helpful with phobias, to decrease anxiety, to allow abreaction or regression, and in the recall of memories in amnesia and fugue states. Hypnosis has been used in substance abuse patients with varying degrees of success. Hypnosis can be used to induce anesthesia for chronic pain, and to permit major surgery without chemical anesthesia.

   Hypnosis is less effective or is contraindicated in patients who have problems with basic trust (paranoid) or who have difficulty in giving up control, as in obsessive compulsive disorder. Patients with phobic and anxiety disorders, hysterical psychosis, and dissociations are highly hypnotizable. Chronic schizophrenics have a lower hypnotizability potential than normal subjects, whereas patients with major affective disorders have a higher potential for hyponotizability than schizophrenics but lower than with normal subjects. (*CTP 1501-16. APA 912-13. Har 210-12.*)

8. (5) A physician's or a therapist's feelings toward a patient may impose a barrier to treatment. The tendency of the physician to displace feelings from earlier figures onto a patient is referred to as countertransference. (See questions 29 and 30 for more details.) (*CTP 1448-49. Har 20, 454.*)

9. (B) Historically, the major figures in developing behavior therapy were Joseph Wolpe (who used Pavlovian techniques, initially with cats, then developed "systematic desensitization," the prototype of many current behavioral procedures), H.J. Eysenck and M.B. Shapiro, and then B.F. Skinner, who developed the "operant-conditioning" model.

   The basic principles of behavior therapy are:
   1. Both normal and abnormal behaviors are learned and maintained in the same ways. Positive reinforcement rewards the behavior, which then occurs more frequently or with greater force. A token economy provides positive reinforcement.
   2. The responses learned from the social environment play a role in the development and maintenance of both normal and abnormal behavior. Therefore, treatment should be preferentially in the natural environment, not in the office.
   3. The major focus of therapy is the behavior problem itself, which is broken up into components that are treated individually through its antecedents and consequences.

4. Behavior therapy is based on a scientific approach.

Behavior therapies consist of the following techniques: systemic desensitization (relaxation training); flooding (see question 10); graded exposure (see question 10); participant modeling (learn by imitating); assertiveness and social skills training; aversive therapy; and positive reinforcements.

"Premack Principle" refers to the observation that habitual or high-frequency behaviors can serve as reinforcers if they are made to follow and be contingent on low-frequency behaviors. (*CTP 262-71, 1462-64. APA 891. Har 551-52.*)

10. **(A)** Behavior therapy in the treatment of agoraphobia uses the techniques of graded exposure and flooding. Flooding is based on the premise that escaping an anxiety-provoking experience (e.g., agoraphobia) reinforces the anxiety through conditioning: by not allowing escape from intense anxiety-provoking stimuli, conditioned avoidance behavior is avoided and anxiety can be prevented.

Graded exposure is similar to flooding except the phobic situation or object is approached through a series of small graduated steps of exposure and is more often carried out in a real-life context. (*CTP 1465-66. APA 892-94. Har 546.*)

11. **(C)** A learned response can be extinguished by reciprocal inhibition where the negative reaction of anxiety is inhibited by an induced or taught relaxed state. Reciprocal inhibition is used in systematic desensitization, and is also referred to as counterconditioning. If a patient attains a state of complete relaxation and then is exposed to the stimulus that usually elicits the feared, anxiety-provoking response, the anxiety is likely to be reduced or extinguished. (*CTP 262-71, 1482. APA 892-94.*)

12. **(D)** Cognitive therapy is a method of brief psychotherapy developed by Aaron Beck, who used "schemes" to describe stable cognitive patterns that the subject uses to interpret experiences. It is based on the premise that normal reactions are mediated by cognitive processes that enable a person to perceive reality accurately. In psychopathology, this ability is impaired and errors in cognition are made. Cognitive therapy is applied mainly to depression (with or without suicidal ideation), panic attacks, obsessive compulsive disorder, paranoid disorders, and somatoform disorders. (*CTP 1549. APA 869-76. Har 536-40.*)

13. **(B)** The cognitive model of depression proposes that symptoms of depression are the result of characteristic distortion in thinking. This consists of a negative self-percept, a tendency to experience the world as negative, demanding, and self-defeating, and an attitude wherein the individual expects failure, punishment, continued hardship, suffering, and deprivation. (*CTP 1542-43. APA 869-70. Har 330-31.*)

14. **(A)** Family therapy involves the treatment of two or more generations together. Couple therapy deals with the resolution of shifting interactions between supposed equals, whereas family therapy has a fixed hierarchy and an expectation of triangles leading to a complex set of problems of structure.

Various founders of schools of family therapy are Nathan Ackerman, Virginia Satir, Carl Whitaker, Murray Bowen, and Ivan Boszormenyi-Nagy. Family therapy using a psychoeducational model can be effective when a family member has a psychosis, depression, or mania. Family therapy is also useful when a child has a conduct disorder or temper tantrums.

Important transactional mechanisms seen in family therapy are:

Double binding—conflicting, inescapable communications

Pseudomutuality—appearance of a sense of relationships to cover underlying conflicts, tensions, lack of valid real relationships

Pseudohostility (converse of pseudomutuality)—appearance of hostility masks underlying anxiety related to intimacy and affection (*CTP 1534-41. APA 935-48. Har 475-77.*)

15. **(B)** See question 9 reference behavior therapy. (*CTP 1462. APA 891. Har 551-52.*)

16. **(C)** The inclusion goals for group therapy are: the ability to perform the group task; problem areas are compatible with the goals of the group; motivation to change. The ideal person for group therapy is similar to that for individual therapy. The subject should be relatively healthy, neurotic, and nonnarcissistic and functioning well socially. Group therapy can also be used with patients who are psychotic, depressed (do better after trusting relations established with therapist), narcissistic, paranoid, or manic (after control by medication). There are few contraindications to group therapy. Some antisocial patients do not adhere to group standards. Delusional patients may incorporate the group in their delusions. Patients who pose a physical threat to others are usually not suitable. Groups for schizophrenics tend to be more supportive than intrusive or introspective and more leader oriented than peer oriented. (*CTP 1523, 2088. APA 956. Har 467.*)

17. **(E)** The structural family therapy model (Minuchin) views the family as a single interrelated system with: (1) significant alliances and splits, (2) hierarchy of power, (3) clarity and firmness of boundaries, and (4) family members' tolerance of one another. It uses concurrent individual and family therapy. The therapist organizes the family into subgroups inducing enactments of al-

tered behavior between members. The technique is most helpful with a variety of psychosomatic disorders of children.

Other family therapy models are:

Strategic (Haley, Milan team, Palo Alto group)—Flexibility, clear rules, large behavioral repertoire.

Behavioral-social exchange (Libermann, Patterson, Alexande.)—Maladaptive behavior is not reinforced, adaptive behavior rewarded, exchange of benefits outweighs costs, long-term reciprocity.

Psychodynamic (Ackerman, Boszormenyi-Nagy, Lidz)—Symptoms are due to the family projection stemming from unresolved conflicts and losses in the family of origin. The therapy uses insight and resolution of the conflicts.

Family systems (Bowen)—Concerns working on differentiation of the self from others in the family in order to obtain an intellectual and emotional balance.

Experiential (Satir, Whitaker)—Symptoms are non-verbal messages in reaction to current common dysfunction in system. Therefore, direct, clear communications are essential in treatment. (*CTP 1540. APA 937-38, 940-41. Har 443.*)

18. **(B)** Cotherapists in group or family therapy can complement, support one another, and provide different role models. In addition, the therapist observational range is broadened. A male-female cotherapist combination has unique advantages, in that it recreates a parental configuration, which can increase affective change of group, can show that a male-female partnership can have mutual respect without derogation, exploitation, or sexualizing, and can increase transferential reactions. A cotherapist can support beginning therapists, especially in helping to clarify transference distortions. A disadvantage is that a cotherapist may take a different ideological position so that therapist splitting occurs. (*CTP 1525. APA 965-66. Har 477.*)

19. **(D)** Supportive psychotherapy aims to help the patient to maintain or reestablish the best possible level of functioning given the limitations of the patient's illness, personality, native ability, and life circumstances. The goal of such therapy is to support reality testing and provide ego support. It is usually best for a fairly healthy individual faced with overwhelming crisis, or a patient without major ego deficits.

Supportive psychotherapy is reality based, and uses suggestion, advice, reinforcement, reassurance, cognitive restructuring, and interpretations to strengthen defenses. (*CTP 1459-61. APA 878. Har 463-65.*)

20. **(C)** The psychoanalysis termination phase reactivates the elements of loss, separation anxiety, and premorbid problems, which are worked through differently. (*CTP 1454. APA 857-59.*)

21. **(A)** Supportive therapy leaves intact and strengthens the patient's defenses by using measures such as reassurance, suggestion, inspiration, persuasion, and education. (See question 19 for more details.) (*CTP 1460. APA 878. Har 963-65.*)

22. **(C)** Brief dynamic psychotherapy uses limited insight-oriented techniques as well as limited objectives and number of visits. The patient must be able to engage quickly, terminate in a short period of time, and be able to carry on much of the working through and generalizing of the treatment effects on his or her own. There is a need for high levels of ego strength, motivation, and responsiveness to interpretation. Transference interpretation is important and done early in the process. Sessions usually are from 10-20 visits, ranging from 5 to 40.

Contraindications to this form of therapy would include a serious recent suicidal attempt, drug addiction, chronic alcoholism, incapacitating chronic obsessional and phobic symptoms, and gross destructive acting out. (*CTP 1564-67. APA 866-68. Har 465-67.*)

23. **(A)** Group therapy provides a means for individuals to work together to resolve underlying conflicts, develop maturity and self-sustaining autonomy.

Goals of the various types of groups are:

Supportive groups—better adaptation to environment

Analytically orientated groups—moderate reconstruction of personality dynamics

Transactional groups—alteration of behavior through mechanisms of conscious control

Behavioral groups—relief of specific symptoms

(See question 25.) (*CTP 1520-25. Har 469.*)

24. **(A)** Individual psychotherapy is the basic form of treatment for narcissistic personality disorder. Patients are chronic and difficult to treat. They react constantly to perceived blows to their narcissism or self-esteem with depression and anger. They are competitive with, scornful of, and devalue but also idealize the therapist. Narcissistic, antisocial, histrionic, and borderline personalities often present with similar symptoms. Abrupt termination of treatment by the patient is not uncommon. (*CTP 1372-73. APA 633-34. Har 345-46.*)

25. **(E)** Group therapy techniques utilized are:

Imparting of information—didactic, interpersonal learning

Altruism—help each other, group cohesiveness

Social learning

Imitative behavior

Catharsis—ventilation of emotions

Procedural aids that can be used:

Written summaries—summary of the group process is made to help understand the here and now

Videotaping—teaching, practice, understanding of group therapy

Structured exercises—follow some specific set of orders

(*CTP 1520-29. APA 957, 977-79. Har 468-69.*)

26. **(B)** Most therapists believe groups should be homogeneous to ensure maximum interactions. This grouping decision should be based on clinical needs. Recent research suggests that good sibling and peer relationships are predictive of successful group participation. (*CTP 1523-25. Har 344, 467-68.*)

27. **(A)** In psychoanalysis, the analytic process involves transference and interpretation (including dreams), which must be well timed; countertransference and transference alliance, which is the therapeutic or working alliance; and resistance. Treatment modalities require certain fundamental rules: the patient must be completely honest with analyst; the patient must be willing to use and share free associations; the patient must delay gratifying any instinctual wishes in order to talk about them in treatment (the rule of abstinence). (See questions 29 and 30, reference countertransference.) (*CTP 1450-51.*)

28. **(D)** The therapeutic alliance is between the patient and analyst, a real relationship in which two adults commit themselves to explore the patient's problems, establish mutual trust, and cooperate with each other to achieve realistic goals of cure or the amelioration of symptoms. (*CTP 1449-51. Har 451-52.*)

29. **(A)** Countertransference refers to a broad spectrum of the analyst's reactions to the patient. Countertransference feelings or behavior may interfere with analyst's ability to remain detached and objective so much so that he or she may need further analysis or self-analysis to resolve the conflicts and deal with the countertransference. (See question 30.) (*CTP 1448-49. Har 454.*)

30. **(E)** Countertransference is the displacement onto the patient of attitudes and feelings derived from the therapist's own inner world, including earlier life experiences. It may be used as a valuable clue to the latent meaning of the patients behavior, thoughts, or feelings. It is the therapist's unconscious contact with the patient's unconscious. (See question 29.) (*CTP 1448-49. Har 454.*)

31. **(E)** Psychoanalysis would be indicated for an individual who has primarily an oedipal conflict with internal tensions, and who is psychologically minded. The analytic candidate should be able to experience and observe strong affects without acting out, and have supportive relationships available in both the present and the past. (*CTP 1455. APA 858.*)

32. **(A)** The psychoanalytic process includes transference, interpretations, countertransference, therapeutic alliance, and resistance. (See question 27 for details.) (*CTP 1446-57.*)

33. **(C)** Prerequisites for insight-oriented (expressive) psychotherapy are a relatively mature personality with a capacity for therapeutic alliance, ability to tolerate frustration, adequate motivation, and some degree of psychological mindedness (insight). Supportive (relationship) psychotherapy prerequisites include a capacity for therapeutic alliance, a personality capable of growth, and a reality situation not too unfavorable. (*CTP 1453. Har 459-63.*)

34. **(E)** Free association is a major element in the technique of psychoanalysis. It is difficult to attain, and much work of the therapy is based on identifying those areas of functioning at which free association breaks down (i.e., defenses clinically experienced by the analyst as resistance). The usual setting is for the patient to lie on a couch or sofa, and the analyst sits behind, partially or totally outside the patient's field of vision. This position helps in patient regression, and allows easier focus on free associations. Other elements in psychoanalysis are the therapeutic alliance, neutrality, abstinence, defense analysis, and interpretation of transference. (*CTP 396, 1443. APA 858-59.*)

35. **(C)** Interpersonal psychotherapy treatment is primarily used for depression (unipolar, nonpsychotic depressions) utilizing 12–16 weekly sessions, usually once per week. The techniques used are reassurance, clarifying of feelings, improvement in interpersonal communications, testing perceptions, development of interpersonal skills, plus the use of medication. (*CTP 1559-60, 1571-72. APA 868. Har 459.*)

6

SOMATIC THERAPIES
Psychopharmacology and Electroconvulsive Therapy

DIRECTIONS: Select the best single response for questions 1 through 36.

1. When a patient does not respond to an antidepressant treatment regimen that is usually effective, what is the most common reason?

   1. The drug is being metabolized unusually quickly
   2. The patient is hypothyroid
   3. The patient is noncompliant
   4. The patient is elderly
   5. The patient does not respond to high plasma levels of the medication

2. Which of the following would be appropriate initial treatment for a patient with major depression with psychotic features?

   1. Monoamine oxidase inhibitor antidepressant
   2. Neuroleptic
   3. Tricyclic antidepressant
   4. Lithium combined with tricyclic antidepressant
   5. Psychomotor stimulant

3. Which antidepressant is most likely to cause akathisia, parkinsonism, and tardive dyskinesia?

   1. Phenelzine
   2. Amitriptyline
   3. Trazodone
   4. Amoxapine
   5. Doxepin

4. All of the following are side effects of imipramine at therapeutic doses except:

   1. Orthostatic hypotension
   2. Ventricular arrhythmias
   3. Hand tremor
   4. Constipation
   5. Weight gain

5. Seizures at therapeutic dose levels are most likely to occur with which of the following antidepressants?

   1. Imipramine

2. Trazodone
3. Phenelzine
4. Desipramine
5. Maprotiline

6. Which antidepressant would be most appropriate to use in treating a 52-year-old depressed male with left bundle branch block and prostatic hypertrophy?

   1. Amoxapine
   2. Trazodone
   3. Imipramine
   4. Maprotiline
   5. Desipramine

7. The most dangerous symptom due to tricyclic antidepressant overdose is:

   1. Coma
   2. Recurrent seizures
   3. Renal failure
   4. Cardiac arrhythmias
   5. Hallucinations

8. The ingestion at one time of a ten-day supply of prescribed medication is likely to be life threatening with which of the following drugs?

   1. Haloperidol
   2. Carbamazepine
   3. Amitriptyline
   4. Diazepam
   5. Perphenazine

9. A depressed patient, taking prescribed phenelzine, snorts "a little cocaine," causing a hypertensive crisis. The best emergency treatment would be:

   1. Physostigmine
   2. Tryptophan
   3. α-methyldopa
   4. Phentolamine
   5. Reserpine

10. All of the following statements about monoamine oxidase inhibitors are correct except:

1. Meperidine is liable to cause convulsions and hyperpyrexia
2. Hypertensive crisis treated effectively with reserpine
3. Amphetamines likely to precipitate hypertensive crisis
4. Orthostatic hypotension frequent problem in elderly
5. Produce total suppression of REM sleep

11. Patients using monoamine oxidase inhibitors may experience dangerous symptoms when they ingest all of the following except:

    1. Cold medications
    2. Cocaine
    3. Meperidine
    4. Yeast breads
    5. Aged, ripe cheese

12. All of the following statements about buspirone are correct except:

    1. Does not potentiate effects of alcohol
    2. Full effect in about two weeks
    3. Effective in suppressing benzodiazepine withdrawal symptoms
    4. Restlessness, nervousness are side effects
    5. Low abuse potential

13. Mania may be caused by each of the following medications except:

    1. L-dopa
    2. Bromocriptine
    3. Amphetamine
    4. Cocaine
    5. Dantrolene

14. Seizures occurring at the usual or slightly above usual clinical dose have been reported in which of the following medications?

    1. Trazodone
    2. Amoxapine
    3. Desipramine
    4. Maprotiline
    5. Imipramine

15. The metabolic synthesis of drugs by liver microsomes is increased by all of the following except:

    1. Smoking
    2. Chronic alcohol use
    3. Methylphenidate
    4. Carbamazepine
    5. Testosterone

16. Drugs that commonly cause depression include all of the following except:

    1. Propranolol
    2. Clonidine

3. L-dopa
4. Guanethidine
5. Reserpine

17. Which of the following statements about the use of triiodothyronine in refractory depression is correct?

    1. Improvement only where the patient is hypothyroid
    2. Improvement is independent of thyroid status
    3. Improvement usually takes three weeks or longer
    4. Antidepressant should be stopped prior to thyroid therapy
    5. Ventricular arrhythmias major problem side effect

18. All of the following statements about tricyclic antidepressants are valid except:

    1. Peak plasma level two to six hours after oral administration
    2. Steady-state blood levels occur about one to three weeks after dose change
    3. Amitriptyline is metabolized to nortriptyline
    4. Imipramine loses therapeutic effect at high plasma levels
    5. Low plasma levels may be due to rapid metabolizing of the drug

19. Early manifestations of lithium toxicity include all of the following except:

    1. Convulsions
    2. Ataxia
    3. Lethargy
    4. Nystagmus
    5. Vomiting

20. All of the following statements about the use of carbamazepine in the treatment of mania are correct except:

    1. Antimanic effect in five to seven days
    2. Aplastic anemia occurs in 1 in 1,000 patients
    3. May produce atrio-ventricular heart block
    4. Reduces serum level of coumadin
    5. Diplopia and ataxia at higher doses

21. Which of the following antidepressants has the least anticholinergic effect?

    1. Amitriptyline
    2. Trazodone
    3. Doxepin
    4. Desipramine
    5. Imipramine

22. All of the following statements about patients on maintenance lithium therapy are correct except:

    1. Clinically severe hypothyroidism is uncommon
    2. Lithium-induced hypothyroidism more common in men

3. Hypothyroidism treated by discontinuing lithium
4. Hypothyroidism treated with thyroid supplement
5. Hypothyroidism more common with prior thyroid dysfunction

23. Appropriate management of lithium toxicity could include all of the following except:

1. Repeated hemodialysis
2. Gastric lavage with activated charcoal
3. Active hydration
4. Cardiac monitoring
5. Chlorothiazide

24. All of the following statements about neuroleptics are correct except:

1. Most antipsychotic medications lower the seizure threshold
2. Acute dystonic reactions tend to occur in first week after initiation or dose change
3. Blurred vision relieved by anticholinergic medication
4. Amantadine used to treat akathisia
5. Acute dyskinesis more common with high-potency neuroleptics

25. All of the following statements about akathisia are correct except:

1. Motor restlessness may be confused with agitation
2. Not caused by inner anxiety
3. Propranolol may produce symptomatic relief
4. Improved by increasing antipsychotic dose
5. Amantadine often therapeutic

26. Which of the following hormones are often increased during antipsychotic drug treatment?

1. Follicle stimulating hormone
2. Testosterone
3. Prolactin
4. Luteinizing hormone
5. Thyroid stimulating hormone

27. A 35-year-old male with delusions of persecution is diagnosed as having paranoid schizophrenia. He is started on thiothixene 5 mg by mouth twice a day and his delusions clear. He is then begun on benztropine 2 mg orally twice daily because of increasing muscle rigidity. After one week on this combined treatment, his wife complains that he appears to be increasingly confused, has lapses of recent memory, and is complaining of seeing things that are not there. Your best treatment procedure would be:

1. Increase thiothixene to 10 mg orally twice a day
2. Increase benztropine to 2 mg orally three times a day
3. Change thiothixene to thioridazine 25 mg twice daily
4. Discontinue benztropine, start amantadine
5. Discontinue thiothixene

28. A 38-year-old woman, agitated and paranoid, is diagnosed as having paranoid schizophrenia. She is started on chlorpromazine 200 mg three times a day by mouth with good symptomatic improvement. After four weeks' treatment, she consults her physician with complaints of tiredness, chills, dry mouth, and throat ulcers. The medication side effect most likely to cause this clinical state would be:

1. Neuroleptic malignant syndrome
2. Agranulocytosis
3. Chlorpromazine jaundice
4. Laryngeal dystonia
5. Anticholinergic toxicity

29. Benzodiazepine receptor sites are most closely related to the receptors for which neurotransmitter?

1. Serotonin
2. Dopamine
3. Gamma-amino-butyric acid
4. Homovanillic acid
5. Acetylcholine

30. All of the following statements about chlordiazepoxide are correct except:

1. Metabolized by glucuronide conjugation
2. Active metabolites
3. Half-life greater than 24 hours
4. Poorly absorbed by intramuscular route
5. Disulfiram increases plasma levels

31. All of the following statements about patients receiving alprazolam are correct except:

1. Abrupt withdrawal liable to cause seizures
2. Less likely to develop dependence, due to drug's short half-life
3. Likely to require multiple doses daily
4. May develop hypomanic behavior dyscontrol
5. Panic attacks may reemerge after medication is withdrawn

32. All of the following statements about tardive dyskinesia are valid except:

1. Involuntary movements may worsen temporarily after stopping neuroleptics
2. Movements are likely to be temporarily reduced if neuroleptic is increased
3. May show improvement if neuroleptic dose is reduced
4. Antiparkinsonian medication produces no benefit
5. Does not occur in schizophrenia patients who have not been given neuroleptics

33. Which of the following statements regarding psychosurgery in the United States are correct?

1. May be beneficial for patients with disabling obsessive compulsive disorder

2. Decreases or abolishes hallucinations in chronic regressed schizophrenia
3. Used for manics unresponsive to pharmacological treatment
4. Effective with chronically suicidal depressed patients
5. Pronounced as unethical by the Task Force of the American Psychiatric Association

34. During electroconvulsive therapy, fasciculations on the chest, abdomen, or foot indicate which of the following?

    1. A subictal response to the electrical stimulus
    2. Depolarizing blocking effect of succinyl choline
    3. Vagal blockage due to atropine
    4. Muscle stimulation effect of short action anesthetic
    5. Underlying anxiety of patient, released by light anesthesia

35. Electroconvulsive therapy is contraindicated in which of the following clinical situations?

    1. Elderly patient with heart block
    2. Middle-aged patient, two months after myocardial infarction
    3. Severely depressed young adult male with frontal lobe glioma
    4. Sixty-year-old female with severe tardive dyskinesia
    5. Twenty-five-year-old woman eight months pregnant with twins

36. Indications for electroconvulsive therapy include all of the following except:

    1. Catatonic schizophrenia not responding to antipsychotic medication
    2. Major depression with persistent suicidal behavior
    3. Severe depression with physical contraindication to antidepressant medication
    4. Obsessive compulsive disorder with severe ritualistic behavior
    5. Schizoaffective disorder not responding to medication

DIRECTIONS: For questions 37 through 95, one or more of the alternatives given are correct. After you decide which alternatives are correct, record your selection according to the following key.

(A) if alternatives 1, 2 and 3 only are correct.
(B) if alternatives 1 and 3 only are correct.
(C) if alternatives 2 and 4 only are correct.
(D) if alternative 4 only is correct.
(E) if all four alternatives are correct.

37. In the management of patients who are not responding to an antidepressant regimen that is usually effective,

which of the following procedures might be appropriate?

1. Try daily triiodothyroninonine 25–50 micrograms
2. Add lithium at low to moderate doses
3. Request plasma drug levels to exclude rapid metabolization
4. Initiate psychotherapy

38. In the management of tricyclic antidepressant overdose, which of the following would be appropriate?

1. Cardiac pacemaker
2. Gastric aspiration
3. Gastric lavage with activated charcoal
4. Renal dialysis

39. Which of the following statements regarding antidepressants are correct?

1. Orthostatic hypotension is a problem with both tricyclic antidepressants and monoamine oxidase inhibitors
2. Imipramine can be used to suppress ventricular irritability
3. Tricyclic antidepressants are contraindicated with preexisting heart block
4. Tricyclic antidepressants can be added to a regimen of monoamine oxidase inhibitors but not the reverse

40. Common side effects of the monoamine oxidase inhibitors include:

1. Orthostatic hypotension
2. Hypomania
3. Impotence
4. Cardiac arrhythmias

41. In panic-prone individuals, which of the following are likely to precipitate panic attacks?

1. Yohimbine
2. Phenelzine
3. Caffeine
4. Clonidine

42. After chronic use, seizures are likely to occur on withdrawal from:

1. Meprobamate
2. Alcohol
3. Diazepam
4. Clozapine

43. Seizures are likely to develop during intoxication with:

1. Cannabis
2. Phencyclidine
3. Lysergic acid diethylamide
4. Cocaine

44. Which of the following statements about liver microsome enzymes are true?

1. Inhibited by cimetidine
2. Inhibited by erythromycin
3. Inhibited by disulfiram
4. Inhibited by barbiturates

45. In the management of a patient who is receiving the anticoagulant warfarin, how would the warfarin dosage have to be adjusted when other medications are added?

1. With phenobarbital, increased warfarin required
2. With carbamazepine, less warfarin needed
3. With disulfiram, less warfarin needed
4. With methylphenidate, increased warfarin required

46. Physostigmine is useful in treating toxicity of:

1. Scopolamine
2. Reserpine
3. Amitriptyline
4. Phenelzine

47. Which of the following statements about clonidine are correct?

1. Reduces symptoms of opioid withdrawal
2. May produce acute hypertension if withdrawn abruptly
3. Can produce depression
4. Gynecomastia is a recognized side effect

48. In which of the following clinical situations would tricyclic antidepressant levels be useful?

1. Possible noncompliance
2. No response to medication dose and duration that are usually effective
3. Patients with marked side effects at low doses
4. Elderly patients

49. When a patient on lithium therapy is treated also with a thiazide diuretic, which of the following statements apply?

1. Increased polyuria
2. Reduction in lithium dose often necessary
3. Higher risk of interstitial nephritis
4. Appropriate treatment for lithium-induced nephrogenic diabetes insipidus

50. With patients on lithium maintenance therapy, which of the following may produce lithium toxicity?

1. Low sodium diet
2. Thiazide diuretics
3. Indomethacin
4. Disulfiram

51. Which of the following commonly occur during lithium therapy?

1. Weight gain
2. Moderate leucocytosis
3. Hand tremor
4. Polyuria

52. Which of the following statements regarding lithium pharmacokinetics are correct?

1. No active metabolites
2. Bound to plasma protein
3. Elimination half-life about 24 hours
4. Therapeutic benefit due to correction of lithium imbalance

53. Which of the following statements about lithium treatment are correct?

1. For acute mania, serum levels 0.8–1.2 mEq per liter recommended
2. Serum levels under 0.5 mEq are ineffective for maintenance therapy
3. With oral administration, peak serum levels occur in two hours
4. Toxicity does not occur with serum levels under 1.5 mEq

54. Which of the following are appropriate treatments for mania?

1. Clonazepam
2. Carbamazepine
3. Valproic acid
4. Electroconvulsive therapy

55. Which of the following statements about the use of carbamazepine in the treatment of mania are valid?

1. Antimanic effect is closely related to electroencephalogram changes
2. Plasma level stabilizes after two weeks' administration
3. Frequent hematological testing reduces risk of hematological reactions
4. May produce false positive pregnancy test

56. In nondepressed patients, imipramine may produce symptomatic benefit in which of the following syndromes?

1. Enuresis
2. Attention deficit hyperactivity disorder
3. Panic disorder
4. Simple phobia

57. Which of the following medications should not be used in combination with tricyclic antidepressants?

1. Propranolol
2. Clonidine
3. Oral anticoagulants
4. Guanethidine

58. Which of the following are side effects of lithium that are likely to occur at therapeutic levels?

    1. Orthostatic hypotension
    2. Flattening or inversion of T waves
    3. Tachycardia
    4. Sinus node dysfunction

59. Which of the following statements about the use of lithium during pregnancy are correct?

    1. When taken during the first trimester, most exposed fetuses have cardiovascular anomalies
    2. Cardiovascular deficits tends to involve the tricuspid valve
    3. Higher level of serum lithium in the fetus as compared with the mother
    4. Lithium in breast milk at concentration half the maternal level

60. Which of the following may cause bucco-lingual masticatory dyskinesia?

    1. Amoxapine
    2. Senile brain changes
    3. Poorly fitting dentures
    4. Metoclopramide

61. A 21-year-old woman is brought to the emergency room. She is restless and confused, feverish and sweating. She complains of stiffness in her face and legs. Her relatives say she has been taking medication for her "nerves," and that evening, she impulsively swallowed pills from the family medicine cabinet when she became upset. Her symptoms could be caused by:

    1. Combined monoamine oxidase inhibitor and meperidine effect
    2. Monoamine oxidase inhibitor–tyramine reaction
    3. Neuroleptic malignant syndrome
    4. Acute neuroleptic toxicity

62. Which of the following statements about agranulocytosis caused by antipsychotic medications are correct?

    1. Usually occurs in the first eight weeks of treatment
    2. Most common in young adults
    3. Mortality rate is often over 10%
    4. Most frequent with high-potency neuroleptics

63. Males on neuroleptic maintenance medication may experience which of the following side effects?

    1. Difficulty achieving an erection
    2. Gynecomastia
    3. Decreased ability to achieve orgasm
    4. Growth retardation

64. Which of the following symptoms are side effects of the neuroleptics?

    1. Amenorrhea
    2. Breast enlargement
    3. Weight gain
    4. Nontoxic goiter

65. Antipsychotic medication causes which of the following side effects?

    1. Paroxysmal tachycardia
    2. Orthostatic hypotension
    3. Hypertensive crisis
    4. Prolonged QT and flattened T waves on the electrocardiogram

66. Which of the following statements are correct about the rabbit syndrome?

    1. Early manifestation of tardive dyskinesia
    2. Treated with anticholinergic medication
    3. Rolling, wormlike tongue movements
    4. Late-onset neuroleptic-induced parkinsonian symptom

67. Plasma antipsychotic levels are decreased by which of the following medications?

    1. Benztropine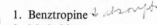
    2. Methyldopa
    3. Barbiturates
    4. Aluminum hydroxide

68. Which of the following statements about dystonic reactions to neuroleptic drugs are correct?

    1. More frequent in young men than elderly women
    2. Laryngeal dystonia may cause ventilation problems
    3. Relieved by intramuscular anticholinergic
    4. Additional anticholinergic often necessary for days after treating initial dystonia

69. When psychotic patients started on 30–60 mg loading doses of haloperidol are compared with those begun on 10 mg per day, which of the following statements apply?

    1. Patients with high loading dose show quicker thought reorganization
    2. Patients on lower initial doses show slower response to treatment
    3. Psychotic symptoms clear more rapidly on higher doses
    4. Patients on higher loading dose develop more dystonias

70. Which of the following statements regarding thioridazine are correct?

    1. Increased Q-R interval and flattened T waves on the electrocardiogram
    2. May cause painful retrograde ejaculation
    3. Dose-related pigmentary retinopathy

4. High incidence of dystonic side effects in young adult males

71. In patients being treated with antipsychotic medication, benztropine is useful in the treatment of:

1. Laryngeal dystonia
2. Blurred vision
3. Rabbit syndrome
4. Tardive dyskinesia

72. Which of the following statements about tardive dyskinesia are correct?

1. Symptoms unaffected by stress
2. Older female patients are more at risk to develop symptoms
3. Improved with bromocriptine
4. Patients with mood disorders are more vulnerable to developing symptoms

73. Which of the following are likely to cause priapism?

1. Trazodone
2. Cocaine
3. Thioridazine
4. Guanethidine

74. Which of the following side effects occur with long-term chlorpromazine use?

1. Purplish gray skin tan
2. Jaundice
3. Lens opacities
4. Retinitis pigmentosa

75. Which of the following medications have active metabolites that are marketed and prescribed?

1. Imipramine
2. Thioridazine
3. Amitriptyline
4. Oxazepam

76. Which of the following medications may result in a false positive or negative dexamethasone test?

1. Indomethacin
2. Estrogens
3. Carbamazepine
4. High-dose benzodiazepines

77. Anxiety symptoms may be produced by which of the following medications?

1. Bronchodilators
2. Nonprescription cold medications
3. Thyroxine
4. Caffeine

78. Drugs that lower the seizure threshold include:

1. Molindone
2. Maprotiline
3. Imipramine
4. Chlorazepate

79. When a patient who has been using benzodiazepines for an extended period is withdrawn from the medication, which of the following statements are correct?

1. Buspirone prevents withdrawal symptoms
2. Severity of withdrawal symptoms is proportional to benzodiazepine dosage
3. Convulsions are more common with sudden withdrawal from long-acting benzodiazepines
4. Reemergence of original anxiety may mimic withdrawal symptoms

80. Which of the following medications have active metabolites?

1. Oxazepam
2. Triazolam
3. Clorazepate
4. Lorazepam

81. If intramuscular benzodiazepine is required, which of the following would be appropriate?

1. Diazepam
2. Alprazolam
3. Lorazepam
4. Clorazepate

82. A 26-year-old chronic schizophrenic is brought to the emergency room because his family states he has been "different." He appears confused and states he does not feel well. He complains that his legs are "not right." His temperature is 37.6 C, his pulse 92, and he is sweating. Possible diagnoses include

1. Drug-induced parkinsonism
2. Acute encephalitis
3. Hypertensive crisis
4. Neuroleptic malignant syndrome

83. Which of the following statements about benzodiazepines are correct?

1. Potentiate the effect of gamma aminobutyric acid
2. Do not cross blood-brain barrier
3. Highly lipophilic
4. Similar pharmacological action to buspirone

84. Which of the following statements concerning long-term antipsychotic therapy are correct?

1. Sexual dysfunction side effects lead to noncompliance
2. May produce male gynecomastia
3. Liable to cause amenorrhea

4. Patients are likely to complain quickly about sexual side effects

85. Which of the following are side effects of lithium?

1. Loss of hair pigmentation
2. Hair loss
3. Hirsutism
4. Exacerbation of psoriasis

86. When unilateral nondominant electroconvulsive therapy is compared with bilateral therapy, which of the following statements are correct?

1. Manic patients respond more completely to unilateral electroconvulsive therapy
2. Once started on unilateral treatment, patients should not be switched to bilateral therapy during a course of treatment
3. Regressed patients show greater benefit from bilateral electroconvulsive therapy
4. Unilateral nondominant treatment causes less amnesia and confusion

87. Which of the following statements about electroconvulsive therapy are correct?

1. For maximum effectiveness, seizures should last 25 to 30 seconds
2. Patient is less likely to have symptom recurrence following electroconvulsive therapy
3. Prolonged seizures tend to produce increased amnesia and confusion
4. Seizure threshold goes down with increasing age

88. Which of the following statements about electroconvulsive therapy are correct?

1. General anesthesia is necessary to allay discomfort of respiratory paralysis
2. Atropine is given to reduce postictal bradycardia
3. Succinylcholine is administered to decrease risk of compression fractures
4. Generalized tonic-clonic seizure is the therapeutic component

89. Prolonged apnea after standard unilateral electroconvulsive therapy may be caused by

1. Barbiturate effect in acute porphyria
2. Inborn deficiency of pseudocholinesterase
3. Cholinergic deficit
4. Acquired enzyme deficiency due to severe hepatic disease

90. Which of the following statements about electroconvulsive therapy are accurate?

1. Contraindicated in patients with severe obstructive pulmonary disease

2. Therapeutic effect in acute mania
3. Mortality rate 0.5 to 1%
4. Depression usually responds to five to ten treatments

91. Which of the following statements regarding amnesia that follows a course of electroconvulsive therapy are correct?

1. Maximum deficits of memory appear immediately after convulsive treatments
2. More frequent treatments cause greater amnesia
3. Amnesia usually clears within two weeks
4. May have permanent amnesia for events during and immediately following treatments

92. Side effects of electroconvulsive therapy include:

1. Amenorrhea for several months
2. Increased high-voltage spiking on the electroencephalogram persisting for one to three months
3. Postictal bradycardia
4. Premature labor

93. Common side effects of fluoxetine include which of the following?

1. Insomnia
2. Leucopenia
3. Diarrhea
4. Weight gain

94. A 37-year-old male chronic schizophrenic patient has not responded clinically to usually adequate doses of standard neuroleptics so you decide to change his medication to clozapine. In discussing possible side effects of this medication with the patient and his family, you will want to point out:

1. Agranulocytosis
2. Seizures
3. Sedation
4. Tardive dyskinesia

95. A 42-year-old depressed female has shown little improvement with phenelzine treatment so you decide to change her medication to fluoxetine. Your treatment plan should be:

1. Over six weeks, gradually decrease phenelzine dosage as you increase the dose of fluoxetine
2. Gradually stop phenelzine over four-week period and then start fluoxetine
3. Maintain phenelzine dosage and start fluoxetine; discontinue phenelzine when fluoxetine dosage has reached usually therapeutic level
4. Wait five weeks after stopping phenelzine before starting fluoxetine

ANSWERS AND EXPLANATIONS

1. **(3)** Noncompliance with prescribed treatment may be due to a denial of the illness, distressing side effects, an unresolved transference to the treatment team, or a delusion that the medication is harmful. Plasma levels can be helpful in determining noncompliance or if there is an unusual metabolism of the drug. (*CTP 1637. APA 796, 1074. Har 509, 530.*)

2. **(2)** A major depression with psychotic features is relatively infrequent, occurring in about 10% of patients with major depression. Delusional depression responds poorly to antidepressants alone: neuroleptics are required with these patients.

   Antidepressants may increase or speed up cycling of recurrent affective disorders. Atypical depressions with symptoms of oversleeping, overeating, mood reactivity, and prominent anxiety may show a preferential response to MAOIs. MAOIs are helpful in depressed females with panic attacks or classic melancholia, whereas depressed males respond better to tricyclic antidepressants. (*APA 792. Har 317.*)

3. **(4)** Antidopaminergic effects such as dystonia, parkinsonism, akathisia, and tardive dyskinesia are rare side effects of antidepressants. However, the active metabolite of amoxapine has dopamine receptor-blocking properties; therefore amoxapine has neuroleptic actions and side effects. (*APA 801. Har 511.*)

4. **(2)** Common side effects of antidepressants, mostly anticholinergic and autonomic symptoms, are dry mouth, sweating, blurred vision, increased heart rate, and impaired conduction, orthostatic hypotension, dizziness or light-headedness (results in falling injuries with elderly), hand tremor, weight gain, and sexual dysfunction. For hand tremor, beta-adrenergic blocking drugs, such as propranolol, have been effective. Imipramine has a quinidine-like antiarrhythmic effect, which may be helpful in treating depressed cardiac patients. (*CTP 1646. APA 799-801. Har 515-17.*)

5. **(5)** The seizure threshold may be lowered by antidepressants. Amoxapine and desipramine have a higher risk of seizures, especially after overdosage, than other antidepressants. A new atypical antidepressant drug, bupropion hydrochloride (Wellbutrin), has a high potential for inducing seizures. (*APA 801. CTP 1647. Har 515-17.*)

6. **(2)** MAOIs do not affect cardiac conduction or rhythm and do not have anticholinergic activity. Trazodone and bupropion have the least anticholinergic side effects of the non-MAOI antidepressants. The antidepressants with high anticholinergic side effects create problems in patients with prostatic hypertrophy or narrow angle glaucoma and should be used with caution, especially in the elderly.

   Amitriptyline (about 5% as potent as atropine) and protryptyline have the highest affinity for the muscarinic receptors, whereas the lowest affinity is with desipramine (1/10th) and trazodone (1/20,000) compared with other tricyclic antidepressants. (*CTP 1645-47. APA 798-801. Har 515, 519.*)

7. **(4)** The cardiac toxicity is due to consequences of the anticholinergic and direct quinidinelike cardiac depressant effects of the tricyclic antidepressants. (See question 4.) Acute hypertensive crisis is potentially the most dangerous effect of MAO inhibitors. (See questions 9 and 11 regarding substances that may precipitate the hypertensive crisis.) (*CTP 1647-48. APA 801-3. Har 515-20.*)

8. **(3)** The tricyclic with the most dangerous side effects and toxicity is amitriptyline because of its anticholinergic properties and effects on the cardiovascular system. (See questions 4, 6, and 7.) (*CTP 1647-48. APA 801-2. Har 515-20.*)

9. **(4)** Patients using monoamine oxidase inhibitor antidepressants are likely to develop a dangerous increase in blood pressure with the concurrent use of tyramine, cocaine, amphetamines, and sympathomimetic amines (e.g., decongestants). Foods that contain large amounts of tyramine (usually more than 10 mg must be ingested to produce hypertension), such as cheese, liver, and yeast extract, must be avoided. (See question 11.) The treatment of this hypertensive crisis is phentolamine (Regitine, an alpha-adrenergic blocker), in doses of 5 mg IV. Narcotic analgesics, especially merperidine (Demerol), are to be avoided in patients taking MAOI due to the risk of hyperpyrexia and seizures caused by an unknown mechanism. (*CTP 1667-68. APA 802-4. Har 515-20.*)

10. **(2)** MAOIs when combined with the acute amine-releasing effects of reserpine or other catecholamine-releasing agents, including guanethidine, can induce a paradoxical hypertensive reaction and cerebral excitation. (See question 9 for treatment of such a reaction.) Antidepressants, including MAOIs, reduce REM sleep and cause hypotension, especially in the elderly. Reserpine is one of the few drugs that increase REM, but it also increases depression. (See questions 4 and 38.) (*CTP 1648-52, 1667-68. Har 519-20.*)

11. **(4)** There is a danger of a serious blood pressure rise when foods containing tyramine are ingested by a patient taking MAOIs. Foods to avoid are aged, ripened cheeses; alcohol (except clear spirits and white wine); yeast extracts; broad beans; smoked or pickled fish; beef

or chicken livers; fermented sausages; and stewed bananas. In addition, medications such as cold remedies, and narcotics such as Demerol, cocaine, amphetamine, sympathomimetic amines, dopamine, and levodopa should be avoided. A tyramine reaction, also called the "cheese reaction," occurs in about 8% of patients on MAOIs who ingest foods or drugs that contain tyramine. Safe foods include yeast (not extract), fresh fruits, fresh cottage cheese, and yogurt. (*CTP 922-23. APA 803-4. Har 519-20.*)

12. (3) Buspirone (BuSpar), an atypical antianxiety agent, has an anxiolytic response different from the benzodiazepines. Buspirone does not interact with other sedative drugs or alcohol. There is no cross-tolerance with benzodiazepines and other sedative-hypnotic drugs such as barbiturates and chloral hydrate. Thus far, there has been no dependence demonstrated, no withdrawal symptoms, no impairment of performance, and no sedation. The full therapeutic action takes about two weeks. (*CTP 1583. APA 812-13. Har 521-22.*)

13. (5) Mania can be caused by many drugs, especially the antidepressants and psychostimulants. (*CTP 631. Har 362-63.*)

14. (4) Maprotiline should be used cautiously in doses above 20 mg/day because of an increased risk of seizures. (See question 5.) (*CTP 1647. APA 801. Har 511.*)

15. (3) Cigarette smoking, chronic alcohol use, carbamazepine, barbiturates, oral contraceptives, and chloral hydrate affect the metabolic breakdown of drugs by interfering with liver microsome enzymes. (See question 57 for more information.) (*CTP 1664-65. APA 802.*)

16. (3) Drugs that commonly cause depression during treatment for a medical condition are:

    Antihypertensives (reserpine, methyldopa, propranolol, clonidine)
    Antiparkinsonians (levodopa, carbidopa, amantadine)
    Hormones (estrogens, progesterone)
    Corticosteroids (cortisone)
    Antituberculosis (cycloserine)
    Anticancer (vincristine, vinblastine)
    (*CTP 631, 901. APA 417.*)

17. (2) The use of triiodothyronine (T$_3$) may potentiate the effects of tricyclic antidepressants in nonresponders. A thyroid profile laboratory study (T$_3$, T$_4$, TSH) should be done to see if subclinical hypothyroidism is present. (*CTP 921. APA 797. Har 514.*)

18. (4) The tricyclic antidepressants are well absorbed after oral administration and do not need to be administered by injection. Plasma concentrations for clinical effec-

tiveness average 100–300 mg/ml. The combined total therapeutic plasma levels for both imipramine and its desmethyl metabolite (desipramine) should be greater than 200–250 ng/ml, with the proportion of desipramine greater than 125 ng/ml. Nortriptyline (metabolite of amitriptyline) has a therapeutic window of 50–150 ng/ml. There are no current levels for MAOIs. (*APA 261-62, 793-94. CTP 1638-42. Har 508-9.*)

19. (1) The general side effects of lithium salts are:
    Hematologic—most frequent leukocytosis (15,000 WBC)
    Parathyroid—increased calcium
    Increased weight gain (frequent)
    Thyroid difficulty (20% hypothyroid)
    Cardiac—suppress function of sinus node ("sick sinus syndrome")
    Skin rash
    Nausea and vomiting (common)

    At mild-to-moderate intoxication levels (1.5–2.0 mEq/l) the following occur:
    Gastrointestinal—vomiting, abdominal pain, dryness of mouth
    Neurological—ataxia, dizziness, slurred speech, nystagmus, lethargy or excitement, muscle weakness

    Moderate-to-severe intoxication (2.0–2.5 mEq/l):
    Gastrointestinal—anorexia, persistent nausea, and vomiting
    Neurological—blurred vision, muscle fasciculation, clonic limb movements, hyperactive deep tendon reflexes, choreoathetoid movements, convulsions, delirium, syncope, EEG changes, stupor, coma
    Circulatory failure—decreased blood pressure, cardiac arrhythmias, conduction abnormalities

    At severe toxic levels (greater than 2.5 mEq/l), generalized convulsions, oliguria, renal failure, and death can occur. (*CTP 1660-61. APA 826. Har 504-7.*)

20. (2) Carbamazepine has been found effective in the treatment of mania, especially in rapid cycling bipolar patients. The effect of carbamazepine is on the kindling phenomenon believed to be causing the rapid cycling. The kindling may be a manifestation of an abnormal limbic neuronal sensitization. Carbamazepine should be started with doses of 200 mg BID and increased by 200 mg/day every five to seven days, to plasma levels of 4–12 μg/ml. A too rapid increase of the drug may produce dizziness, ataxia and anticholinergic blurred vision, constipation, dry mouth, and drowsiness.

    The most serious toxic effect of carbamazepine is aplastic anemia, which may be fatal (rare, occurring in 1/50,000); a more common toxic effect is leukopenia (less than 3,000 WBC), which occurs in about 10% of patients, and thrombocytopenia occurring in 2% of patients. A CBC and platelet count should be done every two weeks at the start of treatment, and then every three months.

Hypersensitivity hepatitis after several weeks of treatment can develop, associated with increased SGOT, SGPT, and LDH. Cholestasis also occurs with increased bilirubin and alkaline phosphatase. Liver function tests SGOT, SGPT, LDH, and alkaline phosphatase, should be done every month at the start of treatment, and then every three months. Other, less common problems are Stevens-Johnson syndrome, hyponatremia (due to the antidiuretic effect), lenticular opacities, and dermatitis. (*CTP 1681-82. APA 827-28. Har 504.*)

21. (2) Antidepressant tricyclics with the least anticholinergic effects are trazodone, fluoxetine, and desipramine, whereas those with the most anticholinergic effects are amitriptyline, protriptyline, trimipramine, and doxepin. (See question 4.) (*CTP 1646. APA 792. Har 515-17.*)

22. (2) During maintenance lithium treatment, hypothyroidism occurs in about 20% of patients and is seen more frequently in women, in patients with thyroid antibodies, and in patients with exaggerated TSH response to TRH. A baseline series of thyroid tests with T_3 (RU), T_4 (RIA), T_4 (free iodine), TSH, and thyroid antibody should be done initially, and then a TSH every six months thereafter.

Treatment for lithium-induced thyroid problems is thyroid replacement 0.05–0.2 mg/day of thyroxine, or reduction or discontinuation of the lithium. As part of the treatment program, other endocrine systems should be checked especially for diabetes mellitus. (*APA 824. CTP 1660-61. Har 506-7.*)

23. (5) When signs of lithium toxicity appear, initially discontinue lithium, increase ingestion of fluids, and do laboratory studies for lithium level, serum electrolytes, and renal function, and an EKG. If toxicity is due to an increased acute ingestion, the initial treatment is gastric lavage and absorption of lithium in the stomach with activated charcoal. Following the lavage, vigorous hydration and maintenance of electrolyte balance are required.

If the serum level is greater than 4.0 mEq/1 within six hours of ingestion, hemodialysis is required and may have to be repeated every six to ten hours until the lithium level is in the nontoxic range and no symptoms of toxicity are present. (*CTP 1660-61. APA 827. Har 504-7.*)

24. (3) The use of neuroleptics can result in many side effects including acute dystonic reactions, parkinsonian syndrome, akathisia, akinesia, rabbit syndrome, tardive dyskinesia, and the neuroleptic malignant syndrome.

Acute dystonic reactions are usually seen within hours or days of the initiation of treatment. Drugs that are used to treat these side effects and other forms of extrapyramidal symptoms produced by blockage of the postsynaptic dopamine receptor are the anticholinergic drugs, dopamine agonists (amantadine, bromocryptine), beta blockers, muscle relaxants (dantrolene), and antidopaminergic drugs (reserpine).

The onset of *parkinsonian syndrome* (or pseudoparkinsonian) and *akinesia* is gradual and occurs usually after weeks.

Akathisia develops shortly after the initiation of treatment, especially with haloperidol.

Rabbit syndrome, perioral tremor, occurs late in treatment.

Incidence of *tardive dyskinesia* increases with age, dose, total time on drug, drug holidays, presence of brain damage, and in those patients with a primary or secondary diagnosis of an affective mood disorder.

Other side effects of neuroleptics are orthostatic hypotension and dizziness, galactorrhea, gynecomastia, amenorrhea, weight gain, decreased libido, pigmentary changes in the eye and skin, arrhythmias, hepatitis, and seizures. (*APA 779-87. CTP 1620-26. Har 492-99.*)

25. (4) *Akathisia* is an extrapyramidal disorder manifested by unpleasant feelings of restlessness and inability to sit still. Akathisia is frequently mistaken for exacerbation of psychotic symptoms, anxiety, or depression. With an increase in medication, there is no improvement of the akathisia and usually there is an exacerbation of symptoms. Decrease in neuroleptic dose may improve the symptoms. Amantadine or beta-adrenergic blocking drugs, such as propranolol, may cause symptomatic improvement, but anticholinergics are usually ineffective in treating akathisia. (*CTP 1624. APA 779-80. Har 492-99.*)

26. (3) During antipsychotic use, prolactin is increased due to the neuroleptic dopamine blocking effects, whereas pituitary gonadotropins (follicle-stimulating hormone and luteinizing hormone) and testosterone decrease. Some reports indicate that amantadine may be effective in the treatment of these hormonal side effects. (See question 25.) (*CTP 1625-26. APA 785-86. Har 498-99.*)

27. (4) *Anticholinergic toxicity* is manifested by restless agitation, confusion, disorientation, tachycardia, dry or flushed skin, dilated pupils, urinary retention, and eventually with more severe toxicity, seizures, hyperthermia, CNS depression, and coma. (*CTP 1622. APA 784-85. Har 494, 516.*)

28. (2) For more information on agranulocytosis, see question 62. (*CTP 1621. APA 787. Har 498-99.*)

29. (3) Benzodiazepine receptor binding sites are intimately linked with the receptor site for gamma-aminobutyric acid (GABA), the major inhibitory neurotransmitter in the brain. Therefore, benzodiazepines potentiate the ef-

fects of the inhibitory action of GABA within the cate-cholamine system. (*CTP 1580-83. APA 806. Har 524.*)

30. (1) Most benzodiazepines, including diazepam, clorazepate, chlordiazepoxide, halazepam, and prazepam, are metabolized by oxidation and hydrolysis to an active desmethylated metabolite. (See answers to question 80.) Drugs such as cimetidine, oral contraceptives, propranolol, disulfiram (Antabuse), and acute alcohol intake inhibit hepatic metabolism, increase the elimination half-life, and increase the half-life of diazepam (normally 60 hours), and chlordiazepoxide (normally 18 hours). (*APA 805-17. CTP 1580-83, 1668. Har 526-27.*)

31. (2) The half-life of alprazolam and lorazepam is 6–12 hours, so more frequent dosing is required with these compounds than the longer acting benzodiazepines. Alprazolam is effective (along with clonazepam) in panic disorder but, after withdrawal and discontinuation of the medication, there can be an increase in anxiety and panic attacks with the occurrence of the medication withdrawal syndrome (malaise, weakness, insomnia, tachycardia, light-headedness, and dizziness). As with any of the benzodiazepines, seizures can occur on abrupt withdrawal. (*CTP 1586. APA 812-16. Har 525-29.*)

32. (5) After symptoms of tardive dyskinesia appear, the only reliable treatment is discontinuing the drug. Even though symptoms can be decreased by increasing the dose of the neuroleptic, symptoms can reemerge in a more severe form. (*CTP 1623-24. APA 781-83. Har 492-99.*)

33. (1) With the introduction of electroconvulsive therapy (ECT) and antipsychotic medication, psychosurgery (leukotomy) fell into disuse. The major indication for psychosurgery is the presence of a debilitating, chronic psychiatric disorder that has not responded to any other treatment. One guideline is that the disorder must have been present for at least three years in spite of many standard treatments having been attempted. Chronic depression and severe obsessive compulsive disorder are the two disorders that have been most responsive to psychosurgery. (*CTP 1679-80. APA 388.*)

34. (2) Succinylcholine, a muscle depolarizing blocking agent, shows initial effect by the development of muscle fasciculations that move in a rostrocaudal progression. The disappearance of these movements indicates that maximal relaxation has been achieved. (See question 88 for more data on ECT.) (*CTP 1671-72. APA 839. Har 580.*)

35. (3) For contraindications to ECT, see question 87. (*CTP 1677. APA 838. Har 584.*)

36. (4) For indications for ECT, see question 87. (*CTP 1676-77. APA 837-38. Har 583-84.*)

37. (E) The physician must try a maximum dose for a minimum of six weeks of tricyclic doses equivalent to 300 mg imipramine, followed by a MAOI dose equivalent to 90 mg phenelzine, before concluding that the depression is refractory to standard pharmacotherapy. Lithium, thyroid hormone (triiodothyronine [T_3]), or psychostimulants can be added to the treatment regimen to promote response. Overall, 70% of depressed patients respond to an adequate trial of medication. (See question 1 regarding noncompliance.) (*CTP 1637. APA 796-98. Har 514-15.*)

38. (A) Tricyclic overdose is treated by gastric aspiration and lavage with charcoal, with close observation for any cardiac toxic effects. The major complications are neuropsychiatric impairment, hypotension, cardiac arrhythmias, and seizures. If the EKG shows a QRS interval less than 0.10, there is decreased likelihood of cardiac problems. If ventricular arrhythmias are present, treatment is with drugs such as lidocaine or propranolol. Death from tricyclic overdose typically occurs within 24 hours of ingestion. With a MAOI overdose, the biggest problem is overstimulation of the sympathetic nervous system. (*CTP 1647-48. APA 801-2. Har 515-16.*)

39. (A) Cardiac effects are common with antidepressants, especially the tricyclics. Orthostatic hypotension is a common, often serious side effect, causing falls and fractures, especially in the elderly. The heterocyclic (especially amitriptyline) antidepressants have more anticholinergic effects than other antidepressants and cause more frequent tachycardias. At therapeutic doses, practically all tricyclics cause prolongation of the PR and QRS intervals. Tricyclic antidepressant should not be used in patients with preexisting heart block. MAOIs and trazodone are relatively free of risk of cardiac conduction abnormalities. EKG monitoring, including ambulatory EKGs if indicated, can be done until a steady state of medication is achieved. Imipramine is a potent antiarrhythmic agent, as it possesses quinidine-like properties. (*APA 799-800. CTP 1644-46. Har 515-17.*)

40. (A) The most frequent side effects of MAOIs are orthostatic hypotension, weight gain, edema, sexual dysfunction, and insomnia. Occasionally there are problems with myoclonus, muscle pains, and paraesthesias. An uncommon side effect is hepatotoxicity. Monoamine oxidase inhibitors have fewer cardiotoxic and fewer epileptogenic effects than the tricyclic antidepressants. Although MAOIs, especially tranylcypromine (Parnate), lack anticholinergic activity, they do have autonomic side effects such as dry mouth and bowel and bladder dysfunction, possibly due to an adrenergic-cholinergic imbalance. (*CTP 1651-52. APA 798-801. Har 517-21.*)

41. **(B)** Lactate infusion will usually precipitate a panic attack in panic-prone patients. The procedure is to use 10 ml of 0.5 molar sodium lactate/kg body weight and infuse over a 20-minute period. About 70–90% of individuals will develop panic attacks if they have a panic disorder, compared with only 0–30% in normal controls. Other panic-inducing agents, carbon dioxide, isoproterenol, beta-carbolene, yohimbine, and caffeine, may be used in diagnostic tests. (*CTP 966. APA 273. Har 237.*)

42. **(A)** Antidepressants, antipsychotics, anxiolytics (benzodiazepines if taken in increased doses over a long period of time), alcohol, and psychostimulants all can lower the seizure threshold and can produce seizures in seizure-prone individuals. (See questions 5 and 78.) (*CTP 1626. APA 801, 815-18. Har 515.*)

43. **(C)** Seizures can occur with lithium overdose, meperidine overdose, phencyclidine and cocaine use as well as with alcohol and barbiturate withdrawal. (*CTP 671-78.*)

44. **(A)** Liver microsome enzymes are inhibited by cimetidine, erythromycin, and disulfiram. (See questions 15 and 57.) (*CTP 1664-65. APA 802.*)

45. **(B)** When the anticoagulant warfarin is used with phenobarbital, increased warfarin is required; but when it is used with disulfiram, decreased warfarin will be needed. (*CTP 1664-65.*)

46. **(B)** Physostigmine and neostigmine are anticholinesterase drugs and can be used to treat an anticholinergic syndrome. They have centrally and peripherally acting reversible anticholinesterase properties and can cause a cholinergic crisis. They are used in the treatment of anticholinergic delirium caused by scopolamine, tricyclic antidepressants, antipsychotics, and other anticholinergic medications. (*CTP 1646. APA 785. Har 498.*)

47. **(E)** Clonidine is effective in treating narcotic withdrawal as it is a nonopioid suppressor of opioid withdrawal symptoms. It may also be effective in treating panic disorder, generalized anxiety disorder, Tourette's disorder (about one-half improve), and ADHD. (*CTP 1683-84. APA 335, 457. Har 711.*)

48. **(E)** Tricyclic blood levels are useful in evaluating compliance in a poor responder to a usually effective dose, side effects occurring at a low dose, potential sensitivity to side effects (as in the medically ill or the geriatric patient), and where therapeutic levels are needed in a short time (as in suicidal patients). (See questions 1 and 18 for blood levels.) (*APA 261-62. CTP 1638-42, 2043-44. Har 508-9.*)

49. **(C)** Most effects of lithium on the kidney are reversible after discontinuing the drug. Lithium causes vasopressin-resistant impairment in renal urine concentration leading to polyuria and nephrogenic diabetes insipidus, and possibly in some patients to tubular interstitial nephritis after long-term treatment. About 60% of patients on lithium complain of increased frequency of urination.

It is important to check renal functions regularly by monitoring BUN (every three to six months), creatinine (if possible, 24 hours urine to measure creatinine clearance), and routine urinalysis. Because of possible hypothyroidism with lithium, thyroid function studies, especially TSH every six months, should be performed. (*APA 822-24. CTP 1661-62. Har 500-1.*)

50. **(A)** Lithium toxicity may be caused by insufficient fluid intake, becoming overheated, sweating excessively, or by excess lithium intake. The patient on lithium must take adequate salt, potassium, and water, especially during hot weather or when exercising. Most diuretics and nonsteroidal anti-inflammatory drugs (NSAIDs), such as indomethacin, but not sulindac, can increase lithium levels. Theophylline increases renal clearance and decreases lithium level. Lithium can cause an increase in the intracellular level of antipsychotic drugs thereby possibly increasing the potential for delirium or the neuroleptic malignant syndrome. There is no interference or change of effect with antidepressants. (*CTP 1669. APA 826. Har 506.*)

51. **(E)** Common side effects of lithium are nausea, diarrhea, polyuria, polydipsia, thirst, fine hand tremor, and fatigue. (In addition, see question 58 for discussion of cardiac effects of lithium.) (*CTP 1660-61. APA 820-25. Har 505.*)

52. **(B)** The precise mechanism of action of lithium is unknown. Multiple intracellular processes are affected by lithium, which inhibits the norepinephrine-sensitive adenylate cyclase, affects the electrolyte balance across the membrane, and reverses or counterbalances many calcium-dependent processes. Lithium is easily absorbed via the gastrointestinal tract and reaches peak plasma levels in one to two hours. The lithium half-life elimination is about 24 hours, so some patients may be maintained on a single daily dose. The steady-state plasma level is reached in about five days. The plasma therapeutic range is 0.8–1.2 mEq/l and should be checked 12 hours after the last dose. (*CTP 1655-56. APA 820. Har 499-501.*)

53. **(B)** See question 52. (*CTP 1655-56. APA 820. Har 500-1.*)

54. **(E)** Treatments used in mania include electroconvulsive therapy, lithium, anticonvulsants (carbamazepine), clonazepam, valproic acid, calcium channel blockers (verapamil), alpha-adrenergic agonists (clonidine), and

beta-adrenergic receptor blockers (propranolol). (*CTP 925-26. APA 819. Har 332-33.*)

55. **(D)** Carbamazepine may produce a false pregnancy test and cause several toxic side effects as noted in question 20. (*CTP 1681-82. Har 333.*)

56. **(A)** Imipramine can also be helpful in panic disorder, as can other drugs such as desipramine and MAOIs phenelzine and tranylcypromine. (*CTP 1835, 1882. APA 792. Har 509-10.*)

57. **(C)** Tricyclic antidepressants are metabolized by hepatic microsomal enzymes. The drugs that should not be used with tricyclics (HCAs) are those that induce hepatic microsomal enzymes, and thus decrease tricyclic plasma levels. The agents that cause this plasma level decrease are alcohol, anticonvulsants, barbiturates, chloral hydrate, glutethimide, oral contraceptives, and cigarettes. Plasma levels of HCAs are increased by antipsychotic drugs, methylphenidate, and aging. The antihypertensive drugs quanethidine and clonidine lose their effectiveness when tricyclics are given at the same time. (*CTP 1669. APA 802. Har 517.*)

58. **(C)** Lithium at therapeutic levels causes flattening or inversion of the T-wave in 20–30% of patients. This EKG change is usually benign. Suppression of the function of sinus node can occur with resultant sino-atrial block or potentially serious aggravation of preexisting ventricular arrhythmias. (*CTP 1661. APA 825. Har 505.*)

59. **(C)** Lithium use during pregnancy, especially in the first trimester, may cause fetal malformations, most often tricuspid valve defects. (*CTP 1659. APA 997. Har 506-7.*)

60. **(E)** Bucco-lingual masticatory dyskinesia is the earliest sign of tardive dyskinesia (involuntary movement of the face, trunk, or extremities) and is usually related to treatment with dopamine-receptor blocking agents. Other drugs, including the antidepressant amoxapine (Asendin) and antiemetic agents metoclopramide and prochlorperazine, and senile brain changes can cause tardive dyskinesia. (*CTP 1623. APA 781-83. Har 496.*)

61. **(B)** *Neuroleptic malignant syndrome* (NMS) is a potentially fatal reaction to antipsychotic agents manifested by severe extrapyramidal effects, lead-pipe muscle rigidity, catatonia, fever and hyperthermia, elevated WBC, tachycardia, abnormal blood pressure fluctuations, tachypnea, diaphoresis, and clouded conscious. Neuroleptic malignant syndrome has been reported more often with the high potency, more frequently prescribed neuroleptics, but can occur with any antipsychotic. Creatinine phosphokinase (CPK) is elevated due to the muscle breakdown (rhabdomyolysis), which may lead to myoglobulinuria (positive for blood in urine, but no

RBCs) and to acute renal failure. (*CTP 1667. APA 783-84, 803-4. Har 495-96.*)

62. **(B)** *Transient leukopenia* (usually a neutrophil count less than 500/ml), and more rarely *agranulocytosis*, is an idiosyncratic reaction to antipsychotic agents. The reaction can occur during the first three or four weeks of treatment, but most often after two to three months of treatment. Periodic blood counts are of no value in predicting occurrence. The overall incidence is less than 0.01% of patients taking antipsychotics. Agranulocytosis is more common in middle age, in females, and with low potency drugs such as chlorpromazine and thioridazine.

Symptoms of leucopenia or agranulocytosis include fever, stomatitis, pharyngitis, lymphadenopathy, and malaise which usually resolve after discontinuing the drug. The mortality rate may be as high as 30% if agranulocytosis is not detected early. Thrombocytopenic or nonthrombocytopenic purpura, hemolytic anemia, and pancytopenia may also occur rarely. (*CTP 162. APA 787. Har 498.*)

63. **(A)** Sexual dysfunctions occur because of the anticholinergic effects, the alpha-adrenergic receptor blockage, and the hormonal effects of the antipsychotic drugs. Males may have difficulty in achieving or maintaining an erection, decreased ability to ejaculate, retrograde ejaculation (especially with thioridazine), and priapism (which requires immediate urological consultation). Females may have changes in quality of orgasm, decreased ability to achieve orgasm, and menstrual irregularities (such as amenorrhea). In both sexes, gynecomastia and galactorrhea causing breast tenderness, decreased libido, and weight gain may occur as side effects. (*CTP 1625-26. APA 785-86. Har 498.*)

64. **(A)** For neuroleptic side effects, see question 24. (*CTP 1625-26. APA 785-86. Har 492-99.*)

65. **(C)** Cardiac side effects include EKG changes of prolonged QT intervals (especially thioridazine), flattened T-waves, and arrhythmias. A serious toxic effect, particular with IM chlorpromazine, would be a sudden suppression of the respiratory system, which can lead to cardiac arrest. Mesoridazine, chlorpromazine, and thioridazine have the most adrenergic side effects, which can cause orthostatic hypotension. (*CTP 1620-21. APA 786. Har 498.*)

66. **(C)** The rabbit syndrome or perioral tremor, an unusual reaction that occurs late, usually after months of neuroleptic treatment, is manifested by fine, rapid movements of the lips that mimic the chewing movements of a rabbit. The syndrome is effectively treated with the anticholinergic drugs or by discontinuing the neuroleptics. (*APA 780-81. CTP 577. Har 495.*)

67. **(B)** Medications that decrease antipsychotic blood levels are, by reducing absorption, antacids, cimetidine, anticholinergics; by increasing metabolism, barbiturates and cigarette smoking. Propranolol increases the blood concentration of neuroleptics. (*CTP 1669.*)

68. **(E)** Acute dystonic reactions can occur within hours to days after initiating neuroleptic treatment. If laryngeal involvement occurs, there may be respiratory and ventilatory distress. The occurrence of dystonias reduces the patient's willingness to continue taking the drugs and the dystonic reaction may interfere with the patient's trust of the physician and confidence in the treatment. The acute dystonic reaction is treated by IV or IM administration of anticholinergic drugs (especially diphenhydramine). This treatment should be followed by the use of oral medications due to the short half-life of the parental drugs. Dystonias are more frequent in patients under 40 years of age, particularly young males. (*APA 779. CTP 1620-26. Har 492-99.*)

69. **(D)** See question 24. (*CTP 1601-2. APA 780. Har 495.*)

70. **(A)** Thioridazine can cause retrograde ejaculation and dose-related pigmentary retinopathy, which can lead to irreversible blindness. (See question 63 and 65 for more details on reactions.) (*CTP 1619-26. APA 779-85. Har 498.*)

71. **(B)** Benztropine (Cogentin), available in oral and parental forms, is used in treating the dystonic reactions, akinesia, parkinsonian syndrome, and the rabbit syndrome. Other drugs that are available to treat extrapyramidal reactions are biperiden (Akineton), diphenhydramine (Benadryl), procyclidine (Kemadrin), and trihexylphenidyl (Artane). (*CTP 1622. APA 780. Har 494.*)

72. **(C)** See question 24 for details about tardive dyskinesias. (*CTP 1623. APA 781-83. Har 492-99.*)

73. **(E)** Priapism can be caused by trazodone, cocaine, thioridazine, and guanethidine. (*CTP 1647.*)

74. **(B)** Long-term treatment with chlorpromazine (or other low-potency high-dose neuroleptics) can cause problems with pigment deposits on the lens, pigmentary retinopathy (especially thioridazine), skin sensitivity to effects of sunlight (especially the aliphatic phenothiazines), and maculopapular eruptions. (*CTP 1625. APA 786-87. Har 492-99.*)

75. **(A)** Active desmethylated metabolites occur with about half of the benzodiazepines and tricyclic antidepressants, but only with a few antipsychotics. The important active metabolites are: imipramine to desipramine; amitriptyline to nortriptyline; thioridazine to mesoridazine; flurazepam to norflurazepam; and diazepam, cloraze-

pate, chlordiazepoxide to oxazepam. (See question 80.) (*CTP 1580, 1639. Har 526-27.*)

76. **(E)** The dexamethasone suppression test (DST) detects abnormalities of the hypothalamic-pituitary-adrenal axis seen in some patients with depression. The procedure is to give the patient dexamethasone 1 mg PO at 11:00 PM; blood is then drawn over next 24 hours at 8:00 AM, 4:00 PM, and 11:00 PM. The test is considered abnormal or positive when the serum cortisol level equals or exceeds 5 μg/dl, depending on local laboratory standards.

Sensitivity for accurately identifying subjects with depression is only 45–50%, whereas specificity (not identifying as positive those who do not have a depression) is 90% in normal subjects, but is less specific with other nondepressed psychiatric patients. Weight loss, medical illnesses (such as diabetes mellitus), medications (steroids, estrogens, phenytoin, carbamazepine, indomethacin, barbiturates), and individual differences in metabolism of dexamethasone can give inaccurate results. (*CTP 531. APA 264-65. Har 134-35.*)

77. **(E)** Commonly used substances producing anxiety symptoms are caffeine, sympathomimetics (over-the-counter medications for colds and allergies), L-dopa, and bronchodilators. Withdrawal from sedatives, hypnotics, and alcohol will produce anxiety symptoms. Physical conditions that manifest anxiety symptoms are hypoglycemia, pheochromocytoma, hyperthyroidism, silent myocardial infarct, pulmonary embolism, small strokes, and cerebral ischemic attacks. (*CTP 968, 1428. APA 273, 1134. Har 237.*)

78. **(A)** Most antipsychotics lower the seizure threshold. Molindone and fluphenazine have the lowest potential to decrease seizure threshold. Antidepressants can lower the seizure threshold, but this is not as marked as with antipsychotics. Bupropion was initially withdrawn from the market because it was reported to increase seizures. Maprotiline has been associated with seizures in therapeutic and toxic doses. Amoxapine and desipramine have a higher risk of seizures after overdose than other antidepressants. (See questions 5 and 42.) (*CTP 1625. APA 787, 801. Har 515-17.*)

79. **(C)** Abrupt withdrawal of benzodiazepines can result in rebound anxiety, and a return of underlying anxiety. If high doses are used, withdrawal symptoms can occur after only six weeks of treatment. It is reported that buspirone has no withdrawal symptoms. Withdrawal symptoms are less severe with long-acting diazepam, but more acute with short-acting alprazolam. (See question 12 regarding buspirone, and 13 for discussion of withdrawal.) (*CTP 1583-86. APA 812-16. Har 521-22, 525-29.*)

80. **(D)** Diazepam, clorazepate, prazepam, halazepam, and flurozepam are metabolized first to desmethyldiazepam

and then follow the same metabolic route as chlordiazepoxide, to oxazepam; thus they have a long half-life. Chlordiazepoxide is metabolized to diazepam, then to desmethyldiazepam, then to oxazepam and finally glucuronide.

Lorazepam, oxazepam, alprazolam, and temazepam have no active metabolites (half-lives of all are from 8–15 hours). Triazolam (Halcion), and some portions of alprazolam, are hydroxylated before going into glucuronidation; therefore triazolam has the shortest half-life of 2–3 hours, whereas the total half-life of alprazolam is 10–15 hours. Imipramine is metabolized to desipramine. (See question 75.) (*CTP 1580-81. APA 812. Har 526-27.*)

81. **(D)** Lorazepam, the only benzodiazepine that has a rapid and reliable absorption by the IM route, is beginning to replace IV diazepam in emergency settings. In the management of PCP intoxication, IV diazepam is still used effectively. (*CTP 1581-82. APA 818-19. Har 526-27.*)

82. **(C)** See question 61 regarding neuroleptic malignant syndrome. (*APA 783-84. CTP 1667. Har 495-96.*)

83. **(B)** Benzodiazepines are lipid soluble so they reach the brain more slowly but maintain blood and brain levels for a longer period of time. (See question 29 referring to GABA.) (*CTP 1580-83. APA 806, 812-16. Har 525-29.*)

84. **(A)** For long-term antipsychotic treatment and side effects, see questions 53 and 74. (*CTP 1619. APA 785-86. Har 492-99.*)

85. **(C)** Side effects of lithium can include acneform follicular eruptions, psoriasis, and skin rash in 7% of patients. Patients on lithium may develop hair changes, including hair loss, thinning, and loss of wave in about 12% of patients, but less so in men. (See questions 50, 51, and 58.) (*CTP 1661-69. APA 825-26. Har 506-10.*)

86. **(D)** Unilateral, nondominant frontotemporal and centroparietal electroconvulsive therapy has fewer adverse cognitive (memory, confusion) effects, but improvement may not be as good as with bilateral, bifrontotemporal electroconvulsive therapy. The use of brief pulse stimulation, instead of sine wave stimulation, can reduce the memory impairment. Retrograde memory loss following bilateral ECT usually clears within six months after treatment.

A generalized tonic-clonic seizure is required for therapeutic effect. An EEG is used to verify the central seizure. Hyperventilation may be needed to induce a seizure. Seizure duration is between 25 and 60 seconds per treatment. With depressed patients, a typical course of ECT consists of six to ten treatments. After ECT treatment, a course of heterocyclic antidepressants or lithium

helps prevent relapse. The role of maintenance ECT is still a matter of controversy.

ECT is generally very safe. The mortality rate is similar to that for general anesthesia, 1/10,000 patients. The most frequent complaints after ECT are memory impairment, headaches, and muscle aches. The most significant risks are cardiovascular with ictal and postictal fluctuations in autonomic tone that can cause cardiac arrhythmias, including premature ventricular contractions, during the immediate postictal period. (See question 87.) (*CTP 1672-73. APA 839. Har 580-81.*)

87. **(B)** The most common indication for electroconvulsive therapy (ECT) is major depression; atypical, neurotic, or reactive depressions do not respond as well. The improvement rate in depressed patients is 80–90%, which is at least equal to or greater than antidepressant medication treatment. ECT is quicker and has fewer adverse effects than drugs. It is the safest treatment in pregnancy, the elderly, and extreme conditions requiring immediate treatment.

Intracranial mass is considered an absolute contraindication, but patients with evolving strokes and recent myocardial infarction pose a high risk. ECT is therapeutic in some types of schizophrenia, especially catatonic and those with a marked affective disturbance, and in mania (particularly acute). (See question 86.) (*CTP 1673-75. APA 839-40. Har 583-84.*)

88. **(E)** Pretreatment procedures required before a course of electroconvulsive therapy (ECT) include a standard physical examination, medical history, blood and urine chemistries, chest X-ray, and electrocardiogram. Spine and skull X-rays, CT scan, MRI, or EEG may be indicated in special circumstances. Prior to the ECT procedure, an anticholinergic agent (such as atropine) is given to minimize secretions and to create a mild tachycardia, which helps prevent treatment-related bradycardia.

The administration of ECT requires general anesthesia, muscular relaxation or paralysis, and oxygenation. Methohexital (Brevital) or thiopental (Pentothal) is used most often for anesthesia. Muscle relaxation drugs such as succinylcholine give adequate relaxation but do not stop all the major ictal body movements. If total relaxation is required, as in musculoskeletal or cardiac disease, IV curare may have to be used. (*CTP 1671-72. APA 839. Har 582.*)

89. **(C)** During electroconvulsive treatments, prolonged apnea may be caused by an inborn or acquired pseudocholinesterase deficiency, or when the metabolism of succinylcholine is disrupted by a drug interaction. (*CTP 1672. APA 839.*)

90. **(C)** See question 86. (*CTP 1670-78. APA 836-40. Har 580-81.*)

91. **(E)** See question 91. (*CTP 1675-78. APA 840-41. Har 582-83.*)

92. **(B)** Memory impairment is related to the amount of electrical stimulation used during the treatments. It is common to have difficulty in remembering events that occurred just prior to the treatment, and difficulty in learning new information immediately after treatment. However, new learning is substantially recovered within six to nine months regardless of whether the patient was given unilateral or bilateral ECT.

Transient cardiac arrhythmias usually occur in patients with existing cardiac disease. The brief postictal bradycardia is usually prevented by increasing the dosage of anticholinergic premedication. The prophylactic use of propranolol is helpful in preventing arrhythmias.

An apneic state may be prolonged if metabolism of succinylcholine is impaired. Toxic side effects or allergic reactions to the pharmacological agents used in the ECT procedure can occur, especially tachycardia from atropine and laryngospasm from anesthetic agents. Fractures and dislocations can result from the induced seizure if musculoskeletal relaxation is not complete. (*CTP 1661-68. APA 840-41. Har 582-83.*)

93. **(B)** Fluoxetine (Prozac), an atypical antidepressant, has selective effects on serotonin by blocking serotonin reuptake. Fluoxetine has a long half-life and can be given in a single daily dose. It causes weight loss rather than weight gain, is not sedating, but rather activates the patient. The commonly observed side effects are nervous system complaints (anxiety, nervousness, and insomnia), drowsiness and fatigue, sweating, gastrointestinal problems (anorexia, nausea, and diarrhea), and dizziness or light-headedness. (*CTP 1631. Har 509.*)

94. **(A)** Clozapine (Clozaril), a dibenzodiazepine, is a potent antipsychotic drug without parkinsonian side effects. Its use was delayed because of the association with agranulocytosis seen in 1–2% of patients at low doses (below 300 mg/day), 3–4% at moderate doses, and 5% at high doses (600–900 mg/day).

Other side effects at regular doses are transient sedation (39%), hypersalivation (31%), tachycardia (25%), constipation (14%), hypotension (9%), hypertension (4%), and weight gain (4%) according to the manufacturer's data. Seizures (3.5–5%) occur at higher doses. Clozapine should not be confused with clonazepam, which is similar to a benzodiazepine and is used for seizure disorders. (*CTP 1626. Har 147, 488.*)

95. **(D)** Fluoxetine has a long half-life and active metabolites. At least five weeks (approximately five half-lives of norfluoxetine) should elapse before starting a MAOI. MAOI should be stopped completely for two weeks before starting fluoxetine. Both procedures are necessary

to avoid the interaction of MAOIs and fluoxetine: death has been reported to occur following the initiation of MAOI therapy shortly after discontinuation of fluoxetine. (*CTP 1631. PDR/90 905-8. Har 509.*)

7

COMMUNITY PSYCHIATRY
Social Psychiatry, Forensic Psychiatry, and Crisis Intervention

DIRECTIONS: Select the best single response for questions 1 through 10.

1. All of the following statements about compliance are correct except:

   1. Compliance is improved when the patient continues to see the same physician
   2. Compliance is better in patients with more chronic illness
   3. Compliance is less in patients who have a multiple dose regimen
   4. Poor compliance may be a direct expression of psychopathology
   5. Compliance is improved with good doctor-patient relationship

2. All of the following statements about postpartum psychosis are correct except:

   1. Peak incidence during first two weeks postpartum
   2. Over 80% are diagnosed as mood disorder
   3. Prophylactic chemotherapy prevents recurrence in most cases
   4. Frequently these patients have obsessive thoughts of harming the infant
   5. Most recover from acute episode

3. All of the following are examples of tertiary prevention except:

   1. Group homes
   2. Social skills training
   3. Genetic counselling
   4. Home visits to monitor medication
   5. Assistance with income support programs

4. All of the following statements about the impaired physician are correct except:

   1. Colleagues tend to deny and cover up the problem
   2. Frequently the physician denies having a problem
   3. Once the physician starts treatment, he or she is likely to persist

   4. Suicide risk higher in male physicians compared with female colleagues
   5. Psychiatrists have significantly higher risk of mood disorder

5. All of the following statements about the psychiatrist expert witness are correct except:

   1. It is unethical to agree on a fee dependent on the trial settlement
   2. It is unethical to rehearse testimony before the court appearance
   3. Psychiatrist has to answer questions even if disadvantageous to his or her client
   4. The judge decides whether the psychiatrist is a qualified expert
   5. The expert is not obliged to answer with "yes" or "no" when asked

6. Recent court decisions regarding involuntary commitment have set the standard of proof of dangerousness as:

   1. 95% certainty
   2. 75% certainty
   3. 51% certainty
   4. 40% certainty
   5. 33⅓% certainty

7. All of the following statements about involuntary commitment are correct except:

   1. Commitment is a legal decision
   2. Commitment has to be to a hospital setting
   3. Commitment usually has a time limit
   4. Commitment is based on the parens patriae principle
   5. Commitment does not require permission of responsible relatives

8. As a result of the California court Tarasoff case rulings, many states have now changed their laws regarding the clinician and:

   1. Criminal responsibility
   2. Threats against a third party
   3. Involuntary commitment

4. Alleged sexual abuse of children

5. Use of hearsay evidence

9. In situations of spouse abuse, all of the following are correct except:

1. Abusing spouse was likely to have been an abused child

2. Abused spouse was likely to have been an abused child

3. Spouse abuse is highly related to drug abuse and alcoholism

4. Pregnancy tends to protect against abuse

5. Abused husbands fear ridicule if they expose the problem

10. In an initial interview, a young male patient becomes increasingly agitated and eventually starts toying with a nasty-looking knife. The clinician, in this situation, could reasonably adhere to any of the following procedures except:

1. Leave the office and call the security staff

2. Offer food to the patient

3. Ask the patient if he wishes medication

4. Ask the patient what is concerning him

5. Insist that the patient hand over the weapon

DIRECTIONS: For questions 11 through 32, one or more of the alternatives given are correct. After you decide which alternatives are correct, record your selection according to the selection key.

(A) if alternatives 1, 2 and 3 only are correct.
(B) if alternatives 1 and 3 only are correct.
(C) if alternatives 2 and 4 only are correct.
(D) if alternative 4 only is correct.
(E) if all four alternatives are correct.

11. Which of the following statements about the mentally retarded in North America are correct?

1. Majority have mild mental retardation

2. Highest incidence of diagnosed retardation in adolescence

3. Most are not diagnosed until they attend school

4. Most eventually require institutional care

12. Examples of secondary prevention include:

1. Establishment of emergency psychiatry clinics

2. Establishment of halfway houses

3. Mandated mental health insurance coverage

4. Vocational rehabilitation programs

13. Examples of primary prevention include:

1. Education about AIDS to high school students

2. Repainting inner-city houses

3. Alcohol abstinence during pregnancy

4. Crisis hotline establishment

14. On which of the following occasions is privileged communication waived?

1. On the decision of the patient

2. On the decision of the physician

3. When the patient is suing the doctor

4. On the decision of the patient's lawyer

15. Which of the following statements about medical privilege are correct?

1. Right of patient to prevent doctor from giving information

2. Obligation of doctor to keep information in confidence

3. Waived when patient's mental status is at issue

4. Physician decides whether to exercise privilege or not

16. Which of the following statements apply to the legal doctrine "Respondeat Superior"?

1. The psychiatrist is legally responsible for the actions of the resident he or she supervises

2. The consultant is usually responsible for the clinical results of the treatment recommended

3. The clinician is obliged to make sure that his or her supervisees live up to accepted psychiatric standards

4. Defines the paternal powers of the state over citizens

17. Which of the following statements about psychiatric expert witnesses are correct?

1. A resident in training cannot be an expert witness

2. Board certification is required for an expert witness

3. An expert witness can only comment on direct observations of the case

4. Testimony of an expert witness may include hearsay evidence

18. Criteria for testamentary capacity include which of the following?

1. Knowledge of one's possessions

2. Knowledge of the natural heirs who would expect to receive bequests

3. Recognition that the individual is making a will

4. Absence of psychotic thinking

19. For a patient to give informed consent, which of the following are applicable?

1. The patient is told about the risks and the benefits of the proposed treatment

2. The patient must give consent willingly and freely

3. The patient knows the alternative treatments possible

4. The patient understands the results of no treatment

20. Which of the following would be appropriate procedures?

1. The patient is discharged from hospital because he refused to consent to a specific treatment
2. The patient is committed because she refused to take medication voluntarily
3. As part of the total treatment, the doctor refused to write to the Social Security office until the patient signed the consent form
4. Because the patient was dangerous to herself, she was legally committed and medication given

21. For a person to be considered competent to stand trial, which of the following should be demonstrated?

    1. Ability to read charges and evidence
    2. Ability to consult with his or her attorney
    3. Ability to know right from wrong
    4. Ability to understand the charges

22. Under the M'Naghten rule, which of the following findings would indicate the individual was not criminally responsible?

    1. The person was involuntarily committed to a psychiatric hospital
    2. The person did not know that the criminal behavior was bad
    3. The individual was mentally retarded
    4. The individual did not understand what he was doing

23. Which of the following statements are correct regarding the M'Naghten rule?

    1. Definition of criminal responsibility
    2. Primarily a test of cognitive functioning
    3. Does not take into account the emotional factors
    4. Focuses on the ability to control impulses

24. The APA statement on the insanity defense makes which of the following points?

    1. Recommends the possible diagnosis "guilty but mentally ill"
    2. Sets out clear guidelines for prediction of dangerousness
    3. Urges reinstatement of the Durham rule
    4. Recommends that psychiatrists evaluate only the patient's mental state

25. Which of the following statements about battered wives are correct?

    1. Pregnancy usually produces reduction in abuse
    2. Much more common among lower socioeconomic groups
    3. Abusing husband usually does not abuse children
    4. Abused wives very often were abused as children

26. In the management of a potentially violent patient, the clinician should use which of the following techniques?

1. Always look the patient directly in the eye
2. Reassure the patient with a gentle pat on the shoulder
3. Interpret the reasons for the patient's feelings
4. Speak in a soft, nonchallenging fashion

27. If a patient produces a gun during an interview, the clinician should take which of the following steps?

    1. Take the gun from the patient
    2. Ask the patient to drop the gun on the floor
    3. Try to ignore the gun and focus on what the patient is saying
    4. Ask the patient to put the gun on the desk

28. Appropriate indications for the use of physical restraints would include which of the following?

    1. Racial insults directed toward staff
    2. Retarded patient threatening other patients
    3. Punishment for repeated stealing from other patients
    4. Delirium of unknown etiology

29. Which of the following statements apply to males who have been raped?

    1. Often fear they will become homosexual
    2. Likely to have post-traumatic stress disorder symptoms
    3. Sexual dysfunction frequent following rape
    4. Feelings of guilt common

30. In the management of a female rape victim, the following procedures are appropriate:

    1. Support the patient in forgetting the trauma
    2. Assistance in reporting the assault to the police
    3. Investigation of previous sexual behaviors
    4. Referral to rape victim group therapy

31. Female rape victims are likely to experience:

    1. Recurrent shame
    2. Feelings of defilement
    3. Fear of male friends
    4. Ruminations about the assault

32. The appropriate emergency management of the female rape victim would include:

    1. Detailed assault report in the patient's own words
    2. Prophylactic treatment for gonorrhea
    3. Collection of pubic hair and vaginal smear specimens
    4. Delayed emotional ventilation until female clinician is available

ANSWERS AND EXPLANATIONS

1. **(2)** Compliance, also called adherence, is the degree to which a patient carries out prescribed treatment. In general, one-third of patients comply, one-third sometimes comply, and one-third do not. There is no association of compliance with the patient's age, sex, marital state, race, or demographic characteristics. Compliance is increased by the physician's characteristics of enthusiasm, permissiveness, age, experience, time spent with the patient, a short waiting time, and the doctor-patient relationship ("match"). Communication is important for the physician to ensure that the patient has a knowledge of the reasons for the treatment, the names of drugs and their side effects, an understanding of the illness, and any compromises made in treatment (patient contract).

   Compliance is decreased if the patient has to take more than three different types of medications and must take them more often than four times a day, utilizing purely verbal instruction if side effects are present, if beneficial effects have slow onset, if the patient has financial hardships or a lack of confidence in treatment, and if there is involvement of multiple clinicians. Psychiatric patients have higher degree of noncompliance than do medical patients. (*CTP 2093-94. Har 411, 530.*)

2. **(3)** About 40–50% of women report "postpartum blues," which is an emotional disturbance or cognitive dysfunction experienced in the postpartum period. Postpartum psychosis is rare, occurring in 1–2 per 1,000 deliveries. Most patients with postpartum psychosis have an underlying mental illness, particularly bipolar disorder, and less often, schizophrenia. A premorbid history of marital problems is also a major factor. Postpartum psychosis occurs usually about the third postpartum day, and most are seen within 30 days. (*CTP 856.*)

3. **(3)** Tertiary prevention is the reduction of the prevalence of a residual defect or disability due to an illness or disorder. It involves rehabilitative efforts to enable those who have a chronic illness, mental or physical, to reach their highest level of functioning feasible. Included in tertiary prevention is a broad range of services such as inpatient, outpatient, and supervised living arrangements; peer, family and community support systems; case management, social and vocational rehabilitation. (*CTP 2069-70. Har 783.*)

4. **(4)** Doctors disabled by alcohol or drugs are often difficult to detect, owing both to the conspiracy of silence surrounding them and their own self-deception. Characteristic behaviors of impaired physicians are first a withdrawal from community and friends; next, change of jobs, often repeatedly; then, their physical status begins to deteriorate; and finally, they can no longer function effectively at office and in the hospital. Those who are involved in rehabilitation programs have a reported 73–97% success rate. (*CTP 1421.*)

5. **(2)** See question 17. (*CTP 2122-23. APA 1064-65.*)

6. **(2)** Involuntary commitment permits hospitalization against a patient's will, is based on the principles of the "parens patriae" (father of the country) and the "police power" of the state, and is justified by an individual's inability to make decisions in his own best interest and the need to protect the individual from himself.

   The minimal legal standard of proof in civil commitment cases is "clear and convincing" of 75% sure, rather than the stricter "beyond a reasonable doubt" of 90% sure for criminal guilt. In civil suits, a "preponderance of the evidence" is based on over 50% certainty and is required for liability. Hearsay is often admissible for involuntary commitment procedures. (*CTP 2115. APA 1071-72. Har 813-14.*)

7. **(2)** Mental health codes' civil commitment laws detail patient's right to treatment and right to refuse treatment. Regulation of commitment is predominantly through statutory law (based on the parens patriae and police power) rather than case law.

   Two legal principles protect all patients against involuntary treatment. The first, from common law, states that a doctor who treats a patient without consent, except under special circumstances (emergency), will be guilty of battery (illegal touching) and the second lays it forth that a doctor who treats a patient without informed consent, except under special circumstances, is guilty of negligence. (See question 19 reference informed consent.)

   The right to treatment is still unsettled in many jurisdictions. The constitutional significance was recognized in Wyatt vs. Stickney (1972), which held: "to deprive any citizen of his or her liberty upon the altruistic theory that the confinement is for humane and therapeutic reasons and then fails to provide adequate treatment violates the very fundamentals of due process." In 1982 (Romero vs. Youngberg), the Supreme Court ruled that the "right to habilitation" was a narrow right to treatment for the institutionalized mentally retarded. (See question 6.) (*CTP 2114-15. APA 1071-73. Har 815-17.*)

8. **(2)** The Tarasoff case (Calif, 1976) set up a standard that applies to a physician or a psychotherapist who has reason to believe that a patient may injure or kill someone. The professional must notify the potential victim, his or her relatives or friends, and the authorities. (*CTP 2119-20. Har 823-25.*)

9. **(4)** See spouse abuse in question 25. (*CTP 1099-1101. APA 642-43.*)

10. **(5)** Offices should not contain heavy throwable objects such as ashtrays, but should contain pillows or a light chair, which can be used as shields or protection. The clinician should communicate in a neutral concrete manner about the obvious, such as "You look angry. Could you tell me what are you concerned about?" The physician should appear calm and in control and speak softly in a nonprovocative and nonjudgmental manner. Undue direct eye-to-eye contact should be avoided. Medications or food can be offered. Continue to evaluate by asking questions. (See questions 26, 27, and 28 for more information on violent patients.) (*APA 1037-55. CTP 1428-33.*)

11. **(A)** For discussions of mental retardation, refer to Chapter 1, Child Psychiatry, and the answers to questions 28, 83, 84, and 86. (*CTP 1728-31. APA 704-5. Har 682-83.*)

12. **(B)** *Secondary prevention* is defined as the early identification and prompt treatment of an illness or disorder with the goal of reducing the prevalence (total number of existing cases) or severity of the condition. The military principles of treatment reference "PIE," Proximity, Immediacy, and Expectancy, could be applied to civilians' programs. Included in secondary prevention strategies are emergency services, outpatient, day treatment, community-based inpatient units, removal of economic barriers to treatment, insurance, and prepaid health plans. (*CTP 2068-69. Har 783.*)

13. **(A)** *Primary prevention* is the prevention of the onset of a disease or disorder thereby reducing its incidence (number of new cases occurring in a specific period of time). Primary prevention strategies include the elimination of etiological agents and reducing risk factors through mental health education, efforts at competence building, development and utilization of social support systems, and anticipatory guidance programs to assist in crisis intervention after stressful events, such as death, marital separation, and group disasters. Other areas of primary prevention include reducing stress during prenatal and perinatal care, by utilizing proper diet, lead pollution laws, and genetic counseling. (*CTP 2068-69. Har 783.*)

14. **(B)** *Privileged communication* refers to the rights of patients that certain confidential information not be disclosed in a judicial setting. Privilege belongs to the patient, not to the physician.

    Confidentiality concerns the communication of private information from one person to another under conditions that the recipient of information will not ordinarily disclose the information to a third person. Con-

fidentiality is limited by legal statute (Tarasoff rule, see question 8).

    Privacy refers to limiting the access of others to one's body or mind, including dreams, fantasies, thought, or beliefs, and is linked to the freedom from intrusion by the state or third persons. (*CTP 2119-20. APA 1088-89. Har 824-25.*)

15. **(B)** Patient information must be kept confidential unless the patient releases the psychiatrist from professional secrecy or else a vital common value in the patient's best interest makes disclosure imperative. The patient must be informed of the breach of secrecy. (See question 14.) (*CTP 2118-20. APA 1088-89. Har 824-25.*)

16. **(B)** The legal doctrine of *"Respondeat Superior"* refers to a physician who supervises another (supervisee) and is responsible both ethically and legally for the quality of the services delivered, due to the actual or apparent control exercised over the supervisee. The supervisor must ensure the patient is informed of such a relationship. (*CTP 2111.*)

17. **(D)** An expert witness provides psychiatric facts or opinions that are relevant to the ultimate legal determination. The expert is required to identify the medical and psychiatric data that are applicable to the existence of a psychiatric disorder and is expected to relate these data to the legal definition of a standard of criminal responsibility. (*CTP 2122-23. APA 1064-65.*)

18. **(A)** Competency to make a will is called *"testamentary capacity"* and cognitive capacity is emphasized. Three psychological abilities are required for individuals to know: (1) the nature and extent of their bounty (property), (2) that they are making a will, and (3) who their natural beneficiaries are. Some additional factors may be used, such as having sufficient mind and memory to understand those facts, ability to recall the decision that was formed, and ability to appreciate the relationship of the facts to one another. (*CTP 2114. Har 820-21.*)

19. **(E)** In general, *informed consent* requires the following criteria or data: (1) the understanding of the nature and the foreseeable risks (side effects) and benefits of a procedure; (2) the knowledge of alternative procedures; (3) the awareness of the consequences of withholding consent; (4) the recognition that the consent is voluntary (no coercion, explicit or implicit); and (5) having the legal capacity to give consent (i.e., adult) and if not, must be a relative or court-appointed guardian. The data should be documented in writing or on a special form. (*CTP 2111-12. Har 817-18.*)

20. **(D)** Involuntary admission is based on evidence that patient is a danger to himself or herself (i.e., suicidal) or a danger to others (homicidal), gravely disabled, and more

recently, a substance abuser. Involuntary admission request may be made by a relative, friend, or police depending on various state legislation. In most states, usually two physicians can hospitalize a patient for up to 60 days, but the patient must have access to legal counsel and a judge to review the case. The patient has a right to file a petition for a writ of habeas corpus by himself, or it can be done by others if it is believed that the patient has been deprived illegally of liberty. Each state has its own standards and procedures for voluntary and involuntary entry into a mental hospital. (*CTP 2111-12. Har 813.*)

21. (C) The test of competency to stand trial is set either by statute or case law and may be worded differently in different jurisdictions. Essentially, competency to stand trial is a two-pronged test involving the capacity to consult with one's lawyer and the ability to understand the proceedings against one. It says nothing of the patient's overall mental competency or functioning. (*CTP 2120-21. Har 806.*)

22. (C) The M'Naghten test (1843) stated that every man is presumed to be sane, and in order to be considered insane, it must be clearly proved that the accused was laboring under such a defect of reason, disease of mind, as to not know the nature and quality of the act he was doing, or, if he did know, that he did not know that what he was doing was wrong. (*CTP 2121. Har 803.*)

23. (A) The M'Naghten test emphasizes cognitive defects and eliminated the requirement to prove frenzy and lack of volitional control. It ignored emotional derangement or loss of volitional control. (*CTP 2121. Har 803.*)

24. (D) Congress adopted in 1982 the definition of insanity based on the American Psychiatric Association and American Bar Association recommendations as to whether the defendant, as a result of mental disease or defect (mental illness), was unable to appreciate the nature and quality of the wrongfulness of his or her conduct (acts), and that "mental illness" was to be limited to a "severely abnormal" mental condition (meaning psychosis). (*CTP 2121-22. Har 805.*)

25. (D) Spouse abuse is a severe problem occurring in every racial and religious group and in all socioeconomic strata. It is more frequent in families of drug abusers, particularly the alcoholic. Men who abuse their spouses generally come from violent homes where they witnessed wife beating or were abused themselves as children. As husbands, they tend to be immature, dependent, nonassertive, and suffer from strong feelings of inadequacy. Wife abuse is most common, but some husbands are abused. Husband abuse is underreported as the men fear ridicule if they expose the problem, counterassault, or loss of financial support. (*CTP 1099-1101.*)

26. (D) Violence and assaultive behavior in a patient are very difficult to predict. The best predictors are excessive alcohol intake, history of violent acts with arrests or criminal activity, and a history of childhood abuse. Violent patients are often frightened by their own hostile impulses and desperately seek help to prevent loss of control. Management of a violent patient is by physical means; restraints should be applied if there is reasonable risk of violence. The patient should be approached with sufficient help and with overwhelming strength, so there is no contest.

Violent, struggling patients may be effectively subdued with appropriate sedative or antipsychotic medication: diazepam (Valium) 5–10 mg (IV), or lorazepam (Ativan) 2–4 mg, IM or IV, haloperidol 5–10 mg IM, or chlorpromazine 25 mg–50 mg IM. The clinician should appear calm and in control, sit if possible, and not tower over the patient. The psychiatrist should listen to the patient and assess violent potential as indicated by threats, availability of means, and history. (See questions 10, 27, and 28.) (*CTP 1427-42. APA 1044-54.*)

27. (D) Safety is the first concern if there is a danger to the therapist. There should be some way to communicate the danger to others, such as a buzzer, code words, or other prearranged signals. If the patient has a gun, comply with requests if one cannot escape. The patient should be asked to put the gun on a desk and not to drop it or throw it as it may discharge. Armed police should always remove bullets from their weapons while in the ER, ward, or clinic. (*APA 1053. CTP 1428-33.*)

28. (C) Emergency seclusion and restraints are used to prevent imminent harm to others or to the patient if other means are not effective or appropriate, to prevent serious disruption of the treatment program or damage to environment (as part of an ongoing behavior treatment program), to decrease stimulation to the patient, and on the patient's request (seclusion). There must be written policy with specific guidance for the staff on the use of seclusion and restraints, with ongoing education, and reviews. (See questions 26 and 27.) (*APA 1044-48.*)

29. (E) Women who are raped experience shame, humiliation, confusion, fear, and rage, lasting a year or longer. Post-traumatic stress disorder, phobia of sexual interactions, and vaginismus are common sequelae. Male rape is legally defined as sodomy. Homosexual rape is more frequent with males. Males feel similar to women who were raped and also feel they "have been ruined" while some fear they will become homosexuals. (*CTP 1099.*)

30. (C) Treatment of rape victims is most effective with immediate support, where the victim is able to ventilate her feelings and rage to loving family members, sympathetic physicians, and supportive law enforcement officials. If the victim knows she has socially acceptable means of

recourse at her disposal, such as arrest and conviction of rapist, this will be therapeutic. Supportive therapy, especially group therapy with homogeneous groups composed of rape victims, is usually beneficial. (*CTP 1096-98.*)

31. (E) See question 29. (*CTP 1098.*)

32. (A) Rape crisis centers and telephone hotlines are available for immediate aid and information for victims. There are legal requirements for the collection of specimens such as pubic hair and vaginal smears for presence of spermatozoa. Trauma to the skin, body, or other activities should be carefully documented with photographs if possible. A detailed report of the incident in the patient's own words should be made as soon as possible in order to prevent later distortions. Prophylactic treatment for venereal disease, such as gonorrhea, is important. (*CTP 1096-99, 1440.*)

APPENDIX

Har 804
Durham test (1954).

An accused is not criminally responsible if his unlawful act was the product of mental disease or mental defect.

Har 804
ALI test (American Law Institute) (1962).

A person is not responsible for criminal conduct if, at the time of such conduct, as a result of mental disease or defect he lacks "substantial capacity" either to appreciate the criminality of his conduct or to conform his conduct to the requirement of law. It is a classic cognitive and volitional test and does not specify the severity or nature of mental diseases, but excludes antisocial personality.

Har 803
Irresistible Impulse Test (1887).

The accused knew right from wrong but, by reason of mental disease, lost power to choose between right and wrong and to avoid doing the act.

8

PSYCHOLOGICAL TESTING

DIRECTIONS: Select the single best response for questions 1 through 6.

1. When a college graduate is asked the meaning of the proverb "people who live in glass houses should not throw stones," her response is "you might get cut by the glass." Her reply shows:

   1. Autistic thinking
   2. Illogical thinking
   3. Concrete thinking
   4. Magical thinking
   5. Abstract thinking

2. A Type I error occurs when:

   1. A null hypothesis is retained when it should have been rejected
   2. A null hypothesis is rejected when it should have been retained
   3. Construct validity is not established
   4. Sample study is not drawn properly
   5. Correlation coefficient is low

3. According to a null hypothesis:

   1. Testing instrument does not measure what it was designed to measure
   2. Risk factor does not precede the disability
   3. Observed differences can be explained by chance alone
   4. Probability rating is zero
   5. Examiners interpret data according to different criteria

4. When a patient scores markedly lower on Block Design and Picture Arrangement Subtests than on Verbal Performance Tests in the Wechsler Intelligence Scale, these results suggest:

   1. Damage to nondominant hemisphere
   2. Major depressive disorder
   3. Malingering
   4. Chronic undifferentiated schizophrenia
   5. Psychogenic amnesia

5. A 35-year-old male, right-handed and moderately aphasic, scores 78 on the Verbal Scale and 99 on the Performance Scale of the Wechsler Adult Intelligence Scale. These test results would support the diagnosis of:

   1. Left hemisphere damage
   2. Bilateral parietal lobe lesions
   3. Right hemisphere damage
   4. Diffuse cerebral deterioration
   5. Conversion disorder

6. In the NIMH Epidemiological Catchment Area studies, the most common disorder, according to one-month prevalence, was:

   1. Obsessive compulsive disorder
   2. Phobia
   3. Dysthymia
   4. Alcohol dependence
   5. Drug dependence

DIRECTIONS: For questions 7 through 27, one or more of the alternatives given are correct. After you decide which of the alternatives are correct, record your selection according to the following key.

(A) if alternatives 1, 2 and 3 only are correct.
(B) if alternatives 1 and 3 only are correct.
(C) if alternatives 2 and 4 only are correct.
(D) if alternative 4 only is correct.
(E) if all four alternatives are correct.

7. Which of the following statements are true about the NIMH Diagnostic Interview Schedule?

   1. Formulated to allow computer scoring
   2. Derived from the Schedule for Affective Disorders and Schizophrenia
   3. Questions are to be read exactly as worded
   4. Developed for nonclinician administration

8. Which of the following statements are true about the Present State Interview?

   1. Used in international studies
   2. Deals mainly with psychoses
   3. Requires specially trained interviewers
   4. Gathers detailed long-range data

9. Short-term memory can be tested by:

   1. Having the patient draw figures after these figures have been removed from view

2. Asking what the patient had for breakfast, when you know the menu
3. Asking the patient to recall five digits reversed
4. Asking who was the first president

10. Which of the following statements about IQ scores on the Wechsler Scale are correct?

    1. 68% of the population have IQ's in the range of 85 to 115
    2. Average IQ is 85 to 100
    3. IQ 110 is at the 75th percentile level
    4. 7% of the population have IQ 70 or below

11. In using the Wechsler Adult Intelligence Scale, early senile dementia should be suspected in a patient where:

    1. Both Visual and Performance scores are lower than premorbid ability
    2. Performance Scale is significantly below Verbal Scale score
    3. Unable to construct blocks to conform to a picture design
    4. Low scoring on Similarities Subtest

12. Serial 7's test:

    1. Is affected by patient's motivation
    2. Measures ability to maintain attention
    3. Is impaired by thought disorder
    4. Errors may indicate depression

13. Correct statements about the Draw-A-Person test include:

    1. Projective test for personality assessment
    2. Intelligence test for children
    3. Can be used to detect brain damage
    4. Better validation than most projective tests

14. When the Bender Gestalt test is used for psychological evaluation, which of the following suggest brain damage?

    1. Language deficits
    2. Perseveration
    3. Color shock
    4. Incomplete angulation

15. Which of the following statements about the Bender Gestalt test are correct?

    1. Designs may be directly copied
    2. Poor motivation may give false positive results
    3. Rotation of figures indicates organicity
    4. Differentiates organic delusional disorders from schizophrenia

16. Which of the following statements about the Rorschach test are true?

1. Ten ambiguous ink blots
2. Each presents black, grey, white, and colored stimuli
3. Sets no limit on number of responses
4. Useful, well-validated research test

17. When the Rorschach test is used to evaluate a patient, which of the following are significant?

    1. The degree to which the patient reacts to the color in the blots
    2. The patient's perception of the actual shape of the blot
    3. The content of the patient's response
    4. The patient's recognition of deviant responses

18. The Rorschach test of an emotionally withdrawn patient will usually demonstrate:

    1. Poor form level
    2. Preoccupation with shades of black and grey
    3. Bizarre content
    4. Few color responses

19. Which of the following statements about the L, F, and K Scales of the Minnesota Multiphasic Inventory are correct?

    1. Useful in identifying malingering
    2. Evaluate attitude toward test-taking
    3. Indicate invalid test if unduly elevated
    4. May be elevated with illiteracy

20. Which of the following statements about the Minnesota Multiphasic Inventory are true?

    1. A series of questions answered true-false
    2. May be computer scored
    3. The most widely researched personality test
    4. Individual clinical scales are specifically diagnostic

21. Which of the following statements about the Thematic Apperception Test are correct?

    1. A series of black, white, and colored pictures
    2. Requires the patient to construct a story
    3. Computer scored
    4. Portrays people in ambiguous situations

22. Which of the following responses on the Rorschach test would support the diagnosis of schizophrenia?

    1. Inability to integrate color into perception
    2. Poor form responses
    3. Contamination of responses
    4. Very limited popular responses

23. In the NIMH Epidemiological Catchment Area Program, studies showed:

    1. Obsessive compulsive disorder higher in men than women
    2. Phobia more common in females than males

    3. Depression more common over age 65 than between ages 25–44

    4. Schizophrenia diagnosed equally in men and women

24. When a test group is said to have normal distribution, which of the following statements would be correct?

    1. 68% of the group lie within two standard deviations of the mean

    2. The median and the mode are equal

    3. The variance is the square root of the standard deviation

    4. The mean and the median are equal

25. In experimental design, which of the following statements are correct?

    1. In normal distribution, two standard deviations from the mean covers 95% of the population

    2. A type 1 statistical error occurs when a null hypothesis is inappropriately retained

    3. A kappa level of 0.80 indicates higher rater agreement

    4. With a normal distribution, the variance and the standard deviation are equal

26. In a research study, which of the following statements are correct?

    1. The independent variable is controlled by the researcher

    2. The dependent variable is the focus of the study

    3. The incidence rate is the rate of new cases occurring within a specific time

    4. ANOVA compares different sets of findings

27. Which of the following statements about the Global Assessment of Functioning Scale are correct?

    1. Rating made for the past six months

    2. Rating 20 would indicate danger to self or others or severe impairment

    3. Includes impairment due to social, physical, and environmental factors

    4. Used on Axis V. of the DSM–III–R

ANSWERS AND EXPLANATIONS

1. (3) The thought content of a patient's thinking can be assessed through responses to various questions obtained during an evaluation. Thought process is the flow of ideas, symbols, and associations. *Normal thinking* is directed toward a reality-oriented conclusion in a logical sequence.

   Autistic thinking has no regard for reality and reveals preoccupations with an inner, private world.

   Illogical thinking contains erroneous conclusions or internal contradictions.

   Concrete thinking is literal and one-dimensional thought with a limited use of metaphors.

   Magical thinking refers to a form of dereistic thought, similar to the preoperational phase in children (Piaget) in which thoughts, words, or actions assume power.

   Abstract thinking is the ability to appreciate nuances of meaning and is multidimensional with the ability to use metaphors and hypotheses appropriately. (*CTP 471–72. APA 188–89. Har 36.*)

2. (2) *Type I* and *Type II errors* are two types of potential errors that can occur in a research or statistical study. A Type I error occurs when the null hypothesis (see question 3) is rejected or declared false when it should have been retained or is true. A Type II error occurs when the null hypothesis is retained as true when it should have been rejected or false. (*CTP 345. APA 73, 1276. Har 48–49.*)

3. (3) The *null hypothesis* is the assumption that there is no significant difference between two random samples of a population. The null hypothesis also states that observed differences or variations in scores can be attributed to random sources. When the null hypothesis is rejected, observed differences between groups are deemed to be improbable by chance alone. (*CTP 354. APA 1275.*)

4. (1) The *Wechsler Adult Intelligence Scale—Revised* (WAIS–R) contains about 80% of the WAIS from the Wechsler-Bellevue series of standardized intelligence tests. There are 11 subtests: 6 in the verbal scale (V), information, comprehension, arithmetic, similarities, digit span, and vocabulary, and 5 in the performance scale (P), digit symbol, picture completion, block design, picture arrangement, and object assembly. Generally the difference between the V and P scales is less than 15 points. Disproportionate impairment in the verbal scale as compared with performance scale is primarily associ-

ated with left (dominant) hemisphere damage and aphasia.

A right (nondominant) hemisphere impairment shows relatively normal verbal scale scores, but marked impairment in the performance scale. A parietal lobe impairment in either hemisphere results overall in a lower performance scale. This pattern is also seen in diffuse cerebral disturbances or in multifocal damage, such as with a head injury or a dementia. A full scale (FS) decrease (both because of verbal and performance lower scores) is seen with depression, poor motivation, and cerebral disease. (*CTP 499. APA 238. Har 50–52.*)

5. (1) See question number 4. (*CTP 499. APA 238. Har 50–52.*)

6. (2) The *NIMH Epidemiological Catchment Area* (ECA) *Study* provides the most complete data about the prevalence of mental disorders in persons of all ages. Results of this study show that about 15.4% of the general U.S. population had one or more DSM–III disorders one month before the interview (males 14% compared with females of 16.6%). Eleven and one-half percent (11.5%) of the population had a substance use problem.

Prevalence rates of other current disorders were: schizophrenia 0.7% (males equal females); affective (mood) disorders 5.1% (males 6.6%, females 3.5%); anxiety (the highest prevalence) 7.3% (females 9.7% much greater than in males 4.7%); phobias (had the greatest increase from prior studies) 6.2%; substance use 3.8% (males 6.3%, females 1.6%); somatization 0.2% (almost all females); antisocial personality disorder 0.5% (males 0.8% and females 0.2%); severe cognitive impairment 1.3% (males equal to females). (*CTP 322–25. APA 82. Har 669–70.*)

7. (E) The *NIMH Diagnostic Interview Schedule* (DIS) was designed for epidemiologic studies of general populations. It combines the Research Diagnostic Interview (RDI) and the Schedule for Affective Disorders and Schizophrenia (SADS). Epidemiologists developed fully structured interviews, according to DSM–III criteria, to be used by nonclinicians to access a large number of subjects. Exact wording is used to each question, with a "yes" or "no" answer. Problems are coded by condition, not by psychiatric illness. The system uses a computer program to score the information and to make diagnostic assignments. The DIS results assess the occurrence of symptoms at any time in the patient's life. (*CTP 317–18, 455. APA 209. Har 767.*)

8. (A) The *Present State Examination* (PSE) measures the current mental state of a patient and is intended for use

by skilled clinicians who are trained in the administration of the test and must demonstrate adequate levels of interrater reliability.

The interview form concentrates mainly on psychotic conditions. Its primary aim was to compare rates of schizophrenia in international studies, and it covers only the one-month state prior to the interview. Historical information is not obtained. PSE results do not give diagnostic labels according to any established classification system. (*CTP 317, APA 78. Har 766.*)

9. (A) *Memory functions* have been traditionally divided into four types: immediate, recent, recent past, and remote. Immediate and recent memory, also called short-term memory, consists of less than five seconds for immediate, and ten seconds to five minutes for recent, and has a capacity limited to about seven, plus or minus two, chunks (or alternatives) of information.

Recent past and remote memory, also called long-term memory, is the retention of experiences over hours or days for recent past, whereas remote goes to earlier life. Long-term memory involves consolidation of information into a relatively permanent store that is subsequently retrievable. (*CTP 502-3. APA 191-92, 1255, 1267. Har 36.*)

10. (B) The Wechsler Scale is designed so that the average performance (average IQ) is a mean of 100 with a standard deviation of 15 points. In addition, norms have been constructed for different age ranges so a subject's IQ can be compared with an age-matched comparison group. The formula for determining the intelligence quota (IQ) is:

$$IQ = \frac{MA \text{ (mental age)}}{CA \text{ (chronological age)}} \times 100$$

The average or normal IQ is 90–110.
IQ of 100 is the 50th percentile.
IQ of 110 is the 75th percentile.
IQ of 90 is the 25th percentile.
68% of population have an IQ of 85–115 (one standard deviation).
95% of population have an IQ of 70–130 (two standard deviations)
(*CTP 497-98. APA 238-39. Har 50-52.*)

11. (E) The Wechsler Adult Intelligence Scale (WAIS) and the WAIS–R have a full scale score (FS) and two major scales, Verbal Scale (VS) and Performance Scale (PS) scores. The Verbal Scale reflects retention of previously acquired (and frequently overlearned) factual information. There are six subtests: Information, Comprehension, Similarities, Arithmetic, Digit Span, Vocabulary.

The Performance Scale measures visuospatial capacity and visuomotor abilities. There are five subtests: Digit Symbols, Picture Completion, Picture Arrangement, Block Design, Object Assembly. When the Per-

formance Scale IQ is significantly lower than the Verbal Scale, this is a useful indicator of cerebral damage. (See question number 4.) (*CTP 498-99, 613. APA 238. Har 50-52.*)

12. (E) Attention and concentration of cognitive functioning can be tested by four tests: Serial 7's, the "A" test, Digit Span, and Spelling Backwards. The Serial 7's test consists of taking 7 from 100 and 7 from each remainder. It requires rudimentary subtraction ability and measures the patient's ability to sustain the task in mind and keep track of sequential answers.

The "A" test consists of the patient tapping his finger every time the examiner says "A." Most individuals can immediately repeat a digit span of at least five digits forward and four digits in reverse order. Most people can spell a five-letter word forward and then backwards. Errors in any of these tests may occur because of poor motivation, delirium, dementia, depression, psychosis, or mental retardation. (*CTP 460. APA 191.*)

13. (A) *Draw-A-Person* (DAP) or Figure Drawings can be classified as projective tests as they allow individuals to project interpersonal, psychic, and familial conflicts or their own personality, onto the drawings. DAP scoring procedures are available for estimation of intelligence and are mostly used with the mentally retarded or with children. A manual is available for dynamic and analytically oriented interpretation of the figure drawings, but such data lack validity. (*CTP 485. APA 363. Har 58.*)

14. (C) The *Bender Gestalt test* consists of nine geometric figures. Some clinicians use the copied figures as a projective test and try to infer personality characteristics, but this use is of questionable validity. The Bender Gestalt test is primarily used as a graphic test for constructional praxis in adults and children since it measures visuoconstructive ability. It can also be used to test memory by waiting 45–60 seconds before having the patient copy the figures from memory. The Bender Gestalt test is helpful in testing for brain damage, where patients are likely to show perseverations, problems with incomplete angulations and juxtaposition, and a tendency to verticalize diagonals, and use substitution of loops for dots. (See question 15.) (*CTP 485, 588f, 1720-21. APA 303. Har 58.*)

15. (A) The Bender Gestalt (Visual Motor) test can be used from ages 3 to 4 years to any older age. There are nine separate designs copied directly on paper. A patient's poor motivation may result in false positives. The rotation of copied figures may indicate organicity. (See question 14.) (*CTP 485, 1720-21. Har 58.*)

16. (B) The *Rorschach (Inkblot) test* is an unstructured, projective test using ten plates of ambiguous inkblots. The patient's responses are scored on multiple criteria refer-

encing accuracy of form, movement, location, use of color, shading, and details; these scores are put into three general coded categories of location, determinants, and form quality content. The test provides information on a patient's level of functioning, maturity, reality testing, interpersonal relations, and emotional responsiveness. It can be helpful in the evaluation of psychosis, suicidality, depression, and anxiety problems. (*CTP 483. APA 234–35. Har 52–54.*)

17. **(E)** The Rorschach results are coded in the following important categories:

location—what portion of blot is utilized
determinants—aspects of blot salient to the patient's perception of form, color, shading, and movement
form content—the specific character of the perception that is human, animal, or nature (See question 16.) (*CTP 483. APA 234–35. Har 52–54.*)

18. **(D)** Rorschach responses of an emotionally withdrawn patient will usually be limited in number, with an avoidance of color responses, and with unimaginative observations. (*CTP 438. APA 234. Har 52–54.*)

19. **(E)** The questions involved in the *Minnesota Multiphasic Personality Inventory* (MMPI) were developed from lists of psychiatric symptoms and complaints and various published personality inventories. The MMPI is a self-report, paper and pencil test, consisting of a series of 550 true-false (T-F) items. The data are shown via three validity scales, and ten standard clinical scales based on norms obtained from large pools of psychiatric and nonpsychiatric clinical patients. The MMPI is set up to assess possible malingering.

The major strength of the MMPI is that it is the most widely used and researched psychological test. Computerized scoring is available. There is a shorter version of the test that consists of 90 items and is used for screening. (*CTP 478–79. APA 229–30. Har 56–57.*)

20. **(A)** See question 19. (*CTP 478–79. APA 229–30. Har 56–57.*)

21. **(C)** The *Thematic Apperception Test* (TAT) started out as a study of normal personalities, but has evolved into a projective test used in psychological examinations. There are 20 cards with pictures varying in content, containing one or more characters, and having various degrees of ambiguity. However, only 10–12 cards tend to be used because of time limitations.

Information is obtained from responses regarding the patient's beliefs, needs, traits, attitudes and motives—in general, a broad spectrum of behavior and cognition. Standardized scoring does exist but most interpretation is impressionistic and informal. (*CTP 483–85. APA 241, 363. Har 54–55.*)

22. **(E)** The Rorschach test has limited value in diagnosing schizophrenia. However, both the Rorschach and TAT responses from psychotic patients generally reveal bizarre ideation. In the Rorschach responses, there is likely to be confabulation and contamination, poorly perceived form responses, repetitions of one concept, a lack of imagination, movement and human content, and an inability to integrate color into the percepts. Overall, there are usually fewer responses and popular observations are often absent. (*CTP 766–67. APA 363. Har 53.*)

23. **(C)** See question 6. (*CTP 322–25. APA 82. Har 669–70.*)

24. **(B)** In a test group, the normal distribution is the mean, median, and mode, and these will be the same when the distribution of scores is normal. The *median* is the halfway point or 50th percentile in the distribution. The *mode* is the most frequent (common) score in the distribution. The *mean* is the arithmetic average and is important in determining the standard deviation. The standard deviation (SD) is a mathematical measure of the spread of scores clustered about the mean. In a normal distribution, 65% of the measurements lie within one SD of the mean, and 95% will be within two SDs of the mean. (*CTP 340–41. APA 1276.*)

25. **(B)** In a population experimental design, a normal distribution consists of 95% of individuals or 2 standard deviations from the average. (See questions 10 and 24.) Kappa (κ) is the most widely used measure of agreement for reliability that corrects for the proportion of chance agreements. Guidelines for interpreting kappa are that values above .75 are excellent, .40–.75 good, and below .40 poor. The value depends on how common the particular condition is in the study sample. (*CTP 313, 340–55. APA 73.*)

26. **(E)** Analysis of variance (ANOVA) is a set of statistical procedures designed to compare two or more groups of observation. The independent variable is studied in relation to an outcome or dependent variable. In experiments, the independent variable is controlled by the experimenter. The dependent variable is the phenomenon of interest in a research study and is also called the outcome variable. The incidence rate is the rate at which new cases of a disease or a condition are occurring within a defined period of time and is usually expressed as a number per 1,000. (*CTP 354. APA 1276.*)

27. **(D)** The *Global Assessment of Functioning* (GAF) is on Axis V of the DSM-III and -III–R Multiaxial System of classification of diagnostic criteria. The summary of the five axes is as follows:

Axis I—Clinical syndromes to include the V codes.
Axis II—Personality and developmental disorders.
Axis III—Existing medical or physical disorders or conditions.

Axis IV—Severity of psychosocial stressors that are relevant to the illness. The rating scale is a continuum of 1 (no stressors) to 6 (catastrophic), and 0 (inadequate information or no change) codes.

Axis V—GAF Scale. The highest level of functioning exhibited during the previous year (social, occupational, and psychological functioning). There is a scale of 1–90, with 1–10 (grossly impaired) to 90 (absent or minimal symptoms, good functioning in all areas) and 0 (inadequate information). (*CTP 465–67. APA 1179. Har 76–79.*)

APPENDIX

CTP 342–46, 354. APA 240. Har 62

TESTS

The T-Test is a statistical procedure designed to compare two sets of observations.

Chi-square (nonparametric statistics) is a set of statistical procedures used to evaluate the relative frequency or proportion of events in a population that falls into well-defined categories.

Variance is an estimate of variability. It is the sum of the squared deviations around the mean, divided by the number of cases.

Standard deviation is the square root of the variance. It gives an estimate of the average deviation around the mean.

The Halstead-Reitan Battery is a neuropsychological test battery consisting of five tests that yield seven summary scores and a total impairment index. The tests contain the following functions: tactile perception, speech sounds, Seashore rhythm, and a finger oscillation test. The battery may take four to six hours to complete. Seashore rhythm test is a nonverbal test for tonal variations developed by Dr. Seashore.

The Luria Nebraska Battery is a neuropsychological test that covers the following 11 areas: motor functions, rhythm skills, tactile and visual functions, receptive and expressive speech, writing, reading, and arithmetic skills, memory, and intelligence.

9
DEFINITIONS

DIRECTIONS: Select the best single response for questions 1 through 28.

1. Primary gain:
   1. Is motivated by pleasure principle
   2. Keeps emotional conflict out of conscious awareness
   3. Is directed by reality principle
   4. Prevents an illness from occurring
   5. Reflects the benefit from being ill

2. "Grass is green. Money is green. Therefore grass is money" is an example of:
   1. Cotard syndrome
   2. Autoscopic phenomenon
   3. Von Domarus principle
   4. Clang association
   5. Pseudologica fantastica

3. Perseveration is the:
   1. Unconscious filling in of memory gaps
   2. Tendency to give same response to different question
   3. Sudden interruption in flow of thought
   4. Repeating back the questioner's words
   5. Incoherent jumble of words

4. Folie à deux is manifested by:
   1. Approximate answers
   2. Claiming a person is an imposter
   3. Taking on the psychosis of another person
   4. Deliberately feigning psychosis
   5. Multiple personalities

5. The unconscious filling in of memory gaps by imagined recollections that the patient believes is called:
   1. Perseveration
   2. Blocking
   3. Derailment
   4. Confabulation
   5. Déjà vu

6. The compulsive handwashing of a guilt-ridden compulsive is an example of:
   1. Undoing
   2. Isolation
   3. Projection
   4. Reaction formation
   5. Displacement

7. A sweet, little old lady has been brought in for examination by the police after they found her wandering through a department store. In response to your question about her address, she replies "State Street" but then in response to the next three questions about other topics, she gives the same answer. Her response is an example of:
   1. Confabulation
   2. Perseveration
   3. Fixation
   4. Circumstantiality
   5. Blocking

8. A newly graduated teacher is finding her new job increasingly difficult. The students are rowdy, the topic she is teaching is unfamiliar to her, and she fears she may be fired. At the start of her second week at work, she tells her supervisor that she is filing a complaint alleging that she is being harassed because she is a woman and a member of a religious minority. Her action may reflect the defense mechanism:
   1. Identification
   2. Splitting
   3. Projection
   4. Malingering
   5. Displacement

9. An 18-year-old woman is brought to the emergency room for examination. She has been a passenger in a car that had been in an accident. Though the car driver was injured, examination shows that the patient has had no physical injury. However, she says that she is "in a fog," and "does not feel right, does not feel real." Her reaction is likely to be an example of:
   1. Post-traumatic stress disorder
   2. La bella indifference
   3. Regression
   4. Dissociation
   5. Depersonalization

10. For the last three months, a middle-aged nurse has noted a gradually enlarging, firm lump in her left breast. When she is asked about this lump at her annual job

physical examination, she answers, "I don't worry about things like that." Her behavior is an example of:

1. Rationalization
2. Denial
3. Regression
4. Displacement
5. Dissociation

11. "If you love me, you will become independent, but if you love me, you will also tell me everything you do," is an example of:

1. Splitting
2. Double bind
3. Isolation
4. Rationalization
5. Undoing

12. When a patient says he experiences red colors everytime he hears a certain sound, this is an example of:

1. Haptic hallucination
2. Synesthesia
3. Cenesthesia
4. Paresthesia
5. Hallucinosis

13. A cocaine abuser complains that "little lice" are crawling over his skin. Repeated physical examinations show no insects on his skin. His complaint is a manifestation of:

1. Cenesthetic hallucination
2. Synesthetic hallucination
3. Haptic hallucination
4. Hypnopompic hallucination
5. Lilliputian hallucination

14. "I feel my brain is burning inside my head" is an example of:

1. Formication
2. Cenesthetic hallucination
3. Autoscopic phenomenon
4. Magical thinking
5. Negative hallucination

15. A 30-year-old married woman is arrested after breaking into the house of a well-known actor. Though this man does not know her, she insists that he is passionately in love with her, is sending her coded messages about his love on television, and wants to be the father of her next child. This woman's behavior is a manifestation of:

1. Propf schizophrenia
2. Munchausen by proxy syndrome
3. Shy-Drager syndrome
4. Scoptophilia
5. Clerembault syndrome

16. An individual who relates to people as if they were all good or all bad is using the mechanism of:

1. Displacement
2. Isolation
3. Projection
4. Splitting
5. Dissociation

17. A 40-year-old man is brought into the emergency room because he attempted to attack his wife. His wife is very concerned, but very supportive. He glares at her and states that, though she looks like his wife in some ways, she is not his wife, but rather someone imitating his wife. The man's behavior is an example of:

1. Cotard syndrome
2. Clerembault syndrome
3. Munchausen syndrome
4. Capgras syndrome
5. Ganser syndrome

18. In dealing with victims of terrorist acts, the Stockholm syndrome may be manifested by:

1. Desire of the victim to testify as to the dedication and kindness of the former captors
2. Recurrent distressing memories of the terrorists' threats
3. Intellectualized discussion of the terrorists' menacing behavior with no outward emotion
4. Wish by the former victims to attack and mutilate the captors
5. Insistence of released victims on returning to their former work even though the risk of kidnapping is still high

19. A 32-year-old man is brought in for examination by the police after he has been accused of shoplifting. The police say the man is confused. In response to your questions, he states his age as 35. His driver's license gives his home street number as 1401, yet he states it is 1302. The day is Friday, but he tells you it is Thursday. His responses are an example of:

1. Witzelsucht
2. Vorbeireden
3. Boufee delirante
4. Verbigeration
5. Merycism

20. "I just lost that thought" would be an example of:

1. Rumination
2. Amnesia
3. Perseveration
4. Blocking
5. Verbigeration

21. Hallucinatory experiences occurring just before full awakening are said to be:

1. Hypnotic
2. Hypnopompic
3. Somnambulism
4. Soporific
5. Narcoleptic

22. A delusion is:

    1. An irrational fear
    2. A misinterpretation of an actual stimulus
    3. A false, fixed belief
    4. A sensory perception without actual external stimulus
    5. A recurrent, unwanted urge to perform an act

23. An example of an illusion would be:

    1. A 46-year-old unmarried woman believing she is the Virgin Mary
    2. A 34-year-old man hearing voices telling him to attack his wife
    3. A 13-year-old girl sure that the shadow in the doorway is a man waiting, as she walks home at night
    4. A 72-year-old man convinced that fire burning in his stomach is destroying his body
    5. A 25-year-old man saying that his wife is not really his wife, but rather is an imposter acting like his wife

24. When asked how a table and chair are alike, a patient states that "they are made of wood." This response is an example of:

    1. Abstract thinking
    2. Flight of ideas
    3. Perseveration
    4. Derailment
    5. Concrete thinking

25. The drift hypothesis is supported by:

    1. Studies that show early onset mental illness leads to lower socioeconomic success
    2. Evidence that schizophrenic patients do not recover fully socially after a psychotic break
    3. Research that indicates that chronic schizophrenics tend to group together
    4. Cognitive studies that demonstrate that the thinking of schizophrenics tends to become more concrete
    5. Biochemical investigations showing increased postsynaptic dopamine receptor blockage with chronic neuroleptic use

26. The defense pattern whereby the emotion related to an idea or concept is made unconscious while the conscious idea remains emotionally bland and no longer anxiety provoking is a characteristic of:

    1. Paranoid disorder
    2. Simple phobia
    3. Somatization disorder

4. Obsessive compulsive disorder
5. Post-traumatic stress disorder

27. The degree to which a test measures what it is intended to measure is its:

    1. Reliability
    2. Sensitivity
    3. Validity
    4. Prevalence
    5. Margin of error

28. A parapraxis may be manifest by:

    1. Sudden thought blocking
    2. Sexual arousal preferentially by nonhuman objects
    3. A slip of the tongue
    4. Insistent, unwanted repetitive urge to do something
    5. Unacceptable behavior symbolically acted out in reverse

DIRECTIONS: For questions 29 through 36, one or more of the alternatives given are correct. After you decide which alternatives are correct, record your answer according to the following key.

(A) if alternatives 1, 2 and 3 only are correct.
(B) if alternatives 1 and 3 only are correct.
(C) if alternatives 2 and 4 only are correct.
(D) if alternative 4 only is correct.
(E) if all four alternatives are correct.

29. According to S. Freud's structural theory, the functions of the ego include:

    1. Adaptation to reality
    2. Regulation of instinctual drives
    3. Development of defense mechanisms
    4. Formation of heterosexual relationships

30. In psychoanalytic structural theory, the superego:

    1. Becomes more punitive as the child moves through the latency period
    2. Is based primarily on the parents' disciplinary style
    3. Is directed by the reality principle
    4. Includes both the conscience and the ego ideal

31. Primary process thinking is:

    1. Mainly verbal
    2. Controlled by regression
    3. Present only in infants and young children
    4. Governed by pleasure principle

32. Examples of secondary gain would include:

    1. Sympathy for being ill
    2. Relief from psychological conflict

3. Freedom to delay difficult decision
4. Minimizing handicapping effect of illness

33. Alexithymia is characterized by:

   1. Expression of emotional feeling through physical sensations
   2. Extensive fantasy
   3. Thinking style similar to Piaget's concrete operations
   4. Unusual ability for empathy

34. A hard-working doctor has to leave his work again to bring home his alcoholic wife. Though she is drunk and dishevelled, gently he helps her clean herself. He prepares a snack for her and then he assists her to her bed. When he returns to the office, his secretary asks if she can leave because it is getting late. He suddenly shouts at her, questioning her efficiency and suggesting that she is neglecting her work. The doctor's behavior indicates he is using which defense mechanisms?

   1. Projection
   2. Reaction formation
   3. Isolation
   4. Displacement

35. Dissociation is a defense associated with:

   1. Alexithymia
   2. Conversion
   3. Hypochondriasis
   4. Fugue

36. In epidemiological studies, the following statements refer to incidence:

   1. Measures occurrence within a definite time period
   2. Indicates population proportion at a specific point in time
   3. Optimally uses at least two examinations of the subjects
   4. Includes all cases occurring during time period

ANSWERS AND EXPLANATIONS

1. **(2)** *Primary gain* is achieved by defense mechanisms that alleviate psychic distress, and the result is a reduction of anxiety and psychological stress. *Secondary gain* is the external gain derived from the symptoms that result in the avoidance of unpleasant situations or responsibility and the attention received from being ill. (*CTP 1013–15. APA 1263, 1267. Har 253.*)

2. **(3)** Illogical thinking contains erroneous conclusions or internal contradictions, and it is only pathological if marked, not in keeping with cultural norms, or is due to an intellectual deficit. (*Har 269. CTP 472.*)

3. **(4)** *Perseveration* is a persisting response to a prior stimulus after a new stimulus has been presented. Perseveration is often associated with organic brain disease. (*CTP 472. APA 1273. Har 39.*)

4. **(3)** *Folie à deux* (or folie à trois), is when two (or three) individuals share the same delusion or communicated emotional illnesses. In DSM-III-R, a disorder of this type is called *induced psychotic disorder.* (*CTP 468. APA 394, 1253. Har 299.*)

5. **(4)** *Confabulation* refers to the fabrication of stories and the unconscious filling of gaps in memory by imagined or untrue experiences that, although the patient believes are true, have no basis in fact. (*CTP 474. APA 1273. Har 95.*)

6. **(1)** *Undoing* is an unconscious defense mechanism where compulsive acts are performed to undo or prevent the consequences or anxiety that the patient irrationally anticipates from a frightening obsessional thought or impulse. (*CTP 988. APA 1270. Har 203.*)

7. **(2)** Perseveration, see question 3; confabulation, see question 5; blocking, see question 20. (*CTP 472, 474. APA 1244, 1273. Har 39, 95.*)

8. **(3)** *Projection* is a defense mechanism operating unconsciously in which the individual attributes (projects) his or her own feelings and wishes to another individual because of intolerable inner feelings or painful affects. (*CTP 375–76. APA 1263. Har 203.*)

9. **(5)** *Depersonalization* is the experience of feelings of unreality or strangeness, such as being detached from one's mental process or body, or a feeling like an automaton, as if in a dream. (*CTP 1038–39. APA 1248. Har 254–55.*)

10. **(2)** *Denial* is a defense mechanism, operating unconsciously, used to resolve or avoid becoming aware of some painful aspects of reality. Denial may be used in a normal state or in a pathological state where it may be replaced as a fantasy or delusion. (*CTP 375. APA 1248. Har 202.*)

11. **(2)** *Double bind* refers to a special form of ambivalence in communication that consists of a simultaneous but mutually contradictory set of directives that assures that the victim will be wrong regardless of which directive is followed and that the victim cannot avoid or escape. (*CTP 581. APA 1249. Har 262.*)

12. **(2)** *Synesthesia* is a sensation or hallucination caused by other sensation modes, such as an auditory sensation triggering a visual sensation. Synesthesia is associated with marijuana, mescaline, and hallucinogen intoxication, or it can occur during a religious experience. (*CTP 474, 571.*)

13. **(3)** A *haptic hallucination* is a hallucination involving touch, such as bugs crawling over skin (formication), and it is common during alcohol withdrawal syndromes and in cocaine intoxication ("cocaine bugs"). (*CTP 571. APA 198. Har 40.*)

14. **(2)** *Cenesthetic hallucination*, also called *somatic hallucination*, is a false sensation of things occurring in or to the body, most often visceral in origin. *Kinesthetic hallucinations* are false perceptions of movement or sensations and commonly occur after the loss of a limb, during toxic states, and in certain schizophrenic reactions. (*CTP 571. Har 40.*)

15. **(5)** *Clerembault's syndrome*, "psychose passionelle," or "erotomania" has been described in two syndromes: (1) a delusional conviction that someone who hardly knows or does not know the patient at all is passionately in love with him or her, and (2) automatisms, explosive and absurd utterances, thought echoes, and a feeling of being possessed and influenced by some dissociated force. (*CTP 458, 851.*)

16. **(4)** In the early stages of ego development, objects are initially divided into good and bad. With increasing ego maturity, the ego is able to synthesize and integrate: the primitive mechanism of splitting is replaced by repression and more efficient defenses. In emotional disorders, such as borderline personality states, splitting is maintained as a primary defense and people are seen as all good or all bad—sometimes the same person on alternate occasions, sometimes different individuals. (*APA 138. Har 187.*)

17. **(4)** *Capgras syndrome*, "illusion de sosies," is a strongly held delusional belief that there are doubles of signifi-

cant others or of oneself, or that the self has been replaced by an imposter. *Fregoli syndrome* is when the patient identifies a familiar person in various other people encountered. *Autoscopic phenomena* are illusions or hallucinations of oneself projected to the outside world. (*CTP 850–51. APA 394. Har 98–99.*)

18. **(1)** Stockholm syndrome takes its name and definition from a hostage situation in Sweden. It occurs during a hostage situation where the victim develops positive feelings toward the captor, usually because the victim is in a situation of total powerlessness, unharmed and released unharmed.

19. **(2)** *Vorbeireden* is a symptom of giving approximate answers or talking past the point, usually ascribed to a factitious disorder, but it can be seen during stress, a fatigue state, or in schizophrenia. Individuals with Ganser syndrome, sometimes termed "syndrome of appropriate answers," respond to simple questions with incorrect answers that indicate that the subject appreciates the correct answer. (*CTP 1139. APA 582. Har 377.*)

20. **(4)** *Blocking* is a term to describe an abrupt interruption or sudden obstruction in spontaneous flow or train of thought and is perceived as an absence or deprivation of thought. Blocking occurs mainly in schizophrenia but may occur in anxiety. (*CTP 472. APA 1244. Har 39.*)

21. **(2)** *Hypnopompic hallucinations* are false sensory perceptions, occurring just before awaking or being fully awake, and are not pathological. *Hypnogogic hallucinations* are false sensory perceptions occurring in healthy people midway between being awake and falling asleep. (*CTP 459, 474, 635. APA 1254. Har 40.*)

22. **(3)** A *delusion* is a false belief based on incorrect inference about external reality and firmly sustained in spite of what is fact. The delusion is strongly held and immutable in the face of refuting evidence. If two share the delusion, the situation is referred to as "folie à deux" (see question 4) and if shared by a family, "folie à famille." (*CTP 563, 817. APA 1248. Har 39.*)

23. **(3)** An *illusion* is a misinterpretation of sensory cues, with a perceptual distortion in estimates of size, shape, and spatial relations. Illusions can occur when one is fatigued or is excessively aroused and can occur with or without a psychiatric disorder. "*Pareidolia*" are voluntary playful and whimsical illusions that occur when one is viewing ambiguous images such as those seen in fire, clouds, patterns in the sand or water.

"*Trailing*" illusions refer to distinct, temporary images of objects seen after the steadily moving objects have already passed. They are usually caused by fatigue, marijuana, or mescaline intoxication. (*CTP 570. APA 1255. Har 40.*)

24. **(5)** *Concrete thinking* refers to literal thinking where there is one-dimensional thought and the limited use of metaphor without understanding of the nuances of meaning. (*CTP 472, 561, 606t. APA 1246. Har 36.*)

25. **(1)** The *drift hypothesis* is based on a type of selection or "drift" of socially incompetent people to the lower classes. (*CTP 302.*)

26. **(4)** According to psychoanalytic theory, patients with an obsessive compulsive disorder use the following defense mechanisms: isolation, undoing, reaction formation, regression, and ambivalence. (*CTP 346. APA 45.*)

27. **(3)** The *validity* of a test refers to the degree to which the test measures what it is supposed to measure.

Reliability is when assessments by the instrument's capacity gives consistent results when used by different examiners at different times (the instrument has acceptable levels of interrating and test-retest reliability).

Sensitivity refers to the measure of an instrument's ability to detect the true cases of a disorder identified by the criterion instrument.

Specificity is the ability to identify true noncases identified by the criterion instrument.

Prevalence refers to the patients who have a disorder at a specified time regardless of how long ago the disorder started. (*CTP 313. APA 227. Har 48–49.*)

28. **(3)** *Parapraxis* is an act, blunder, or lapse of memory, such as a slip of the tongue or pen, or mislaying of objects, usually because of an unconscious motive (according to Freud). (*CTP 1451. APA 1260.*)

29. **(E)** Ego functions (ref. S. Freud) are a substratum of the personality and perform the tasks of mediating between the instincts and the outside world. (*CTP 372–74. Har 178–80. APA 132–35.*) The ego's functional tasks are:
    1. control and regulation of instinctual drives
    2. relation to reality
    3. object relations
    4. synthetic functions of the ego (integrative capacities)
    5. primary autonomous ego functions (perception, intuition, comprehension, thinking, language, motor development, learning, intelligence)
    6. secondary autonomous ego functions
    7. defensive functions of the ego

30. **(C)** The *superego* is the last psychic structure to develop and results from the resolution of and is heir to the Oedipus complex. During latency, the superego internalizes standards, restrictions, and punishments set by the parents and is further modified during the adolescent period. (*CTP 374–77. APA 134. Har 180–81.*)

31. **(D)** *Primary process thinking* is irrational and primary—metaphorically, sometimes called "right-brain" thinking, is associated with visual images and creative thought, and is motivated by the pleasure principle. Primary process thinking uses symbols, metaphor, imagery, condensation, displacement, and concretism. *Secondary process thinking*, or rational thinking, is language-associated thoughts based on reality. It allows one to think abstractly and appreciate complex thought, and the process is predictable, coherent, and redundant. (*CTP 560. APA 126–27. Har 173.*)

32. **(B)** *Secondary gain* represents the tangible benefits received as a result of becoming sick. (See question 1.) (*CTP 1015. APA 1267. Har 13–14.*)

33. **(B)** *Alexithymia* refers to a disturbance in the affective and cognitive functions resulting in a person who expresses very little emotion or fantasy, even in a situation likely to generate strong emotions in most people. It has been suggested that subjects with alexithymia are more likely to express their feelings by somatization. (*CTP 573. APA 1240. Har 390.*)

34. **(C)** *Reaction formation* occurs when an unacceptable impulse is transformed into its opposite. The defense is used at an early stage of ego development and is characteristic of obsessional character states. *Displacement* is a defense mechanism operating unconsciously, where an emotion or drive cathexis from one idea or object is shifted to another object that resembles the original in some aspect or quality but is more acceptable as a focus. This defense permits symbolic representation of the original idea or object to be assumed by another idea or object that is less highly cathected or that evokes less distress. (*CTP 376. APA 1249, 1265. Har 203, 205.*)

35. **(C)** Dissociation occurs when there is splitting off of clusters of mental contents from conscious awareness, and where there is a modification of a person's character or of one's sense of personal identity in order to avoid emotional distress. Fugue states or hysterical conversion reactions are common manifestations of dissociation. (*CTP 376. APA 1249. Har 203, 205.*)

36. **(B)** *Incidence* is the rate of only new cases that come into being during a clearly defined period of time. For a study to be done carefully, at least two examinations of each subject in the sample are needed, one at the start and one at the end of the designated time period. (*CTP 314. APA 1275. Har 762–63.*)

APPENDIX

Clang association (*CTP 458, 472, 561*)—association of words similar in sound but not in meaning, no logical connection, may include rhyming and punning.

Compensation (*APA 1246*)—an unconscious defense mechanism where one attempts to make up for real or fancied deficiencies.

Conversion (*APA 1247*)—an unconscious defense mechanism where intrapsychic conflicts that cause anxiety are given symbolic external expression, especially somatic symptoms involving the central nervous system.

Cotard's syndrome, "delire de negation" (*CTP 458, 851*)—delusions of guilt, or delusions of immortality, poverty, and even nihilism. Common in psychotic endogenous depression.

Déjà vu (*CTP 474*)—illusion in which a new situation is incorrectly regarded as a repetition of a previous event.

Derailment (*CTP 472*)—gradual or sudden deviation in train of thought without blocking. Synonymous with loosening of association.

Idealization (*APA 1254*)—an unconscious or conscious mental mechanism in which one overestimates an admired aspect or attribute of another.

Identification (*APA 1254*)—an unconscious defense mechanism where an individual patterns his or her behavior after some other individual. It is different from the conscious process of imitation or role modeling.

Incorporation (*APA 1255*)—a primitive unconscious defense mechanism in which the psychic representation of a person, or parts of a person, is figuratively ingested.

Isolation (*CTP 987*)—an unconscious defense mechanism in which the affect attached to an idea is rendered unconscious, leaving the conscious idea emotionally neutral and protects individual from anxiety-provoking affects and impulses. Affect and impulse are separated from the ideational component and pushed out of consciousness. Social isolation refers to the absence of object relationships.

Magical thinking (*APA 1257*)—a conviction that thinking and doing are the same. It is characterized by a lack of a real relationship between cause and effect.

Pseudologica fantastica (*CTP 473, 567, 1136–37*)—a type of lying where person believes in the reality of his or her own fantasy and acts on these beliefs.

Rationalization (*APA 1265*)—an unconscious defense mechanism in which an individual attempts to justify feelings, behavior, or motives that otherwise would be intolerable. It is not the same as conscious evasion or dissimulation.

Sublimation (*APA 1268*)—an unconscious defense mechanism where instinctual drives are diverted into socially acceptable behavior.

Symbolization (*APA 1269*)—a general mechanism where some mental representation stands for something else and the link between the symptom and symbol is usually unconscious.

10
CASE HISTORIES

DIRECTIONS: Select the single best response for each of the questions 1–45.

1–4. An 18-year-old woman is brought to evaluation because her parents are concerned about her weight loss in the past year. Since her girlfriends teased her about being "plump," she has been maintaining a strict diet. She used to be slightly overweight at 155 pounds, but now weighs 91 pounds. Her menses started when she was 13 years old, but stopped three months ago. The patient is active and energetic: she considers herself "normal and healthy."

1. The most likely diagnosis is:

   1. Atypical depression
   2. Conversion disorder
   3. Anorexia nervosa
   4. Prader Willi syndrome
   5. Separation anxiety disorder

2. On physical examination, in addition to weight loss, it is likely to be noted that she has:

   1. Fine lanugo hair on both arms and legs
   2. Loss of hair pigmentation
   3. Diminished or absent pubic hair
   4. Masculine pubic and chest hair
   5. Patchy alopecia

3. Laboratory investigations are likely to show:

   1. Elevated T_4 levels
   2. Increased cortisol secretion
   3. Reduced growth hormone
   4. Leucocytosis
   5. Lowered blood urea nitrogen

4. All of the following statements about this disorder are correct except:

   1. Poorer prognosis with late onset
   2. Greater risk of suicide when binge and purge
   3. Occurs primarily in upper socioeconomic groups
   4. Less than 10% occur in males
   5. Higher incidence of mood disorders in first-degree relatives

5–6. A 26-year-old man has been suffering from recurrent disabling diarrhea for two years. Repeated extensive studies have given marginally abnormal or normal results. All treatments have been ineffective. The young man and his family insist that "something has to be done," but the patient is annoyed when psychiatric consultation is recommended because, "I'm not crazy."

5. As the next stage in this patient's management, it would be appropriate to do:

   1. Fecal testing for phenolphthalein
   2. Amytal interview
   3. MMPI for evidence of malingering
   4. Repeat colonoscopy
   5. Laparotomy

6. Your further procedure confirms your diagnosis of which of the following syndromes?

   1. Cotard
   2. Munchausen
   3. Capgras
   4. Da Costa
   5. Clerembault

7–8. You are called in consultation regarding a 45-year-old man with a 16-year history of bipolar disorder. In recent years, his affective symptoms have been well controlled with lithium. He has had occasional stomach discomfort and a slight bilateral hand tremor. Routine testing, however, has shown his serum lithium level to be 1.9 mEq per liter.

7. You advise:

   1. Discontinue lithium
   2. Check creatinine clearance
   3. Request thyroid stimulating hormone level
   4. Repeat lithium level 12 hours after last dose
   5. Change medication to carbamazepine

8. The patient asks how the effect of lithium might change as he gets older. You tell him all of the following except:

   1. With increasing age, lithium has decreasing therapeutic effect
   2. Older patients require lower dosage of lithium
   3. Lithium has longer half-life in elderly
   4. Serum level 0.4 mEq per liter often effective in older patients
   5. Lithium may exacerbate psoriasis

9–12. A 6-year-old boy is referred for evaluation because he does not sit still in class, constantly interrupts the other students, and will not pay attention to the class work. He is an active youngster at home, often up early in the morning, watching television and playing with his dog.

9. His mother brings him for examination, but he starts to cry when he is asked to come to the interview playroom. You should:

    1. Insist that the child come with you by himself
    2. Cancel the interview and tell them to return when the child is less fearful
    3. Interview mother and child together for a few minutes and then ask the mother to leave
    4. Interview mother and child together for the complete examination
    5. Interview the boy in the waiting room

10. As you watch mother and patient together, you note that he is affectionate and polite. He is occasionally restless, but he stays on his chair for the ten-minute wait. Based on your initial observation and history, your probable diagnosis is:

    1. Separation anxiety disorder
    2. Mild mental retardation
    3. Pervasive developmental disorder
    4. Attention deficit hyperactivity disorder
    5. Oppositional defiant disorder

11. Treatment for this patient could include all of the following except:

    1. Pemoline
    2. Imipramine
    3. Phenobarbital
    4. Methylphenidate
    5. Dextroamphetamine

12. All of the following statements about this disorder are correct except:

    1. Onset usually in preschool years
    2. Diagnosed most often in grade school period
    3. Symptoms will clear with onset of adolescence
    4. Increased incidence of adult antisocial behavior
    5. Higher incidence in patients with Tourette's disorder

13–14. A 28-year-old unmarried woman is referred for psychiatric evaluation prior to surgery because of reportedly recurrent mood swings. She has already had two laparotomies for abdominal pain and her gall bladder was removed elsewhere. Her family suspects that she must be using drugs because, at times, she appears to be "almost confused."

13. Which test would you recommend?

    1. Serum folate
    2. Urinary methemoglobin
    3. Serum phosphokinase
    4. Serum bilirubin
    5. Urinary porphobilinogen

14. Appropriate management of this patient would include all of the following except:

    1. Avoid alcohol
    2. Oral contraceptives to regulate menses
    3. Low-dose chlorpromazine for pain
    4. Discontinue barbiturates
    5. Carbohydrate loading during acute episodes

15–19. A 52-year-old woman comes to the emergency room seeking "side effect medication." She has a 30-year history of chronic undifferentiated schizophrenia with multiple past hospitalizations. In recent years, she has been maintained on oral low-dose haloperidol with good symptom control. She now states that she feels "bad." Her jaws and arms are stiff, her temperature is 38C, her blood pressure 140/100, and her white cell count 20,000.

15. Which one laboratory test would you request first?

    1. Hepatitis antigen
    2. HIV antibodies
    3. Serum creatine phosphokinase
    4. Serum aspartate aminotransferase
    5. Blood urea

16. While you await the test result, you would:

    1. Stop haloperidol
    2. Stop haloperidol, change to clozapine
    3. Continue haloperidol, start amantadine
    4. Stop oral haloperidol, start depot haloperidol
    5. Continue present oral haloperidol

17. Which of the following diagnoses is likely to be correct?

    1. Neuroleptic-induced parkinsonism
    2. Incipient catatonia
    3. Early tardive dyskinesia
    4. Viral encephalitis
    5. Neuroleptic malignant syndrome

18. Treatment of this syndrome is likely to include:

    1. Doxepin
    2. Disulfiram
    3. D-penicillamine
    4. Bromocriptine
    5. Pyridoxine

19. The patient and her family emphasize that haloperidol has successfully controlled her symptoms unlike other neuroleptics tried. You advise them:

    1. Restarting haloperidol will cause symptoms to recur
    2. Haloperidol can be restarted at a lower dose with careful monitoring to see if symptoms recur
    3. This syndrome occurs only with haloperidol
    4. Depot medication does not cause this syndrome
    5. This syndrome shows a strong family incidence

20–22. For three weeks a 26-year-old woman has been increasingly disruptive. She has been claiming that she is a famous rock star and has been staying up all night singing and dancing. She has been argumentative and threatening with her family. Though she appears increasingly tired physically, she continues to be constantly active.

20. Emergency management of this patient could include all of the following except:

    1. Haloperidol
    2. Lorazepam
    3. Hypnosis
    4. Physical restraints
    5. Electroconvulsive therapy

21. Eventually you decide that lithium would be the preferred maintenance treatment for this patient. Before you start lithium therapy, all of the following tests are required except:

    1. Pregnancy test
    2. Electrocardiogram
    3. Electroencephalogram
    4. Serum creatinine
    5. Thyroid function

22. You alert the patient and her family to the common side effects of lithium, which include all of the following except:

    1. Weight gain
    2. Hair loss
    3. Hypotension
    4. Diarrhea
    5. Polyuria

23–25. A 6-year-old girl has been investigated for repeated hematuria. This symptom has recurred over the past nine months. Typically, the patient is admitted to the hospital after several days gross hematuria. With rest alone, the symptom clears quickly and the child appears to be healthy. Soon after return home and the resumption of activities, the hematuria recurs. Multiple investigations have given normal or equivocal results. With her latest bout of hematuria, it was found that the blood in the patient's urine did not match the patient's blood type.

23. The likely diagnosis is:

    1. Capgras syndrome
    2. Father-daughter incest
    3. Precocious puberty
    4. Munchausen by proxy syndrome
    5. Acute intermittent porphyria

24. In these clinical situations, the involved parent is usually:

    1. Physically abusive toward the patient
    2. Solicitous and attentive to the patient
    3. Cold and emotionally distant
    4. Inadequate and overwhelmed
    5. Bizarre and unpredictable

25. A further evaluation of the involved parent is likely to demonstrate symptoms of:

    1. Schizophrenia
    2. Personality disorder
    3. Mental retardation
    4. Masked depression
    5. Multiple personality

26–30. A 55-year-old female physician is hospitalized with a fractured femur following a car accident. Four days after hospital admission, she is noted to be tachycardiac, restless, sweating, and fearful. She is bothered by what she describes as "vague shapes," which she sees coming out of the walls.

26. As you take a more detailed history from her husband, you anticipate that he will describe symptoms in his wife of:

    1. Bipolar disorder
    2. Recurrent schizophrenia
    3. Chronic alcohol abuse
    4. Histrionic personality disorder
    5. Acute intermittent porphyria

27. Your treatment recommendations could include all of the following except:

    1. Magnesium sulfate
    2. Thiamine
    3. Chlordiazepoxide
    4. Chlorpromazine
    5. Parenteral fluids

28. Two weeks later, her acute symptoms have subsided. Though you have never treated her before, she talks with pleasure about the many years, she says, you have cared for her and her family. She is now manifesting symptoms of:

1. Korsakoff's syndrome
2. Malingering
3. Folie à deux
4. Pathological intoxication
5. Bouffee delirante

29. Neuropathological examination of patients with these symptoms typically shows:

    1. Hepatolenticular degeneration
    2. Pontine hemorrhages and necrosis
    3. Hemorrhages and sclerosis of mammillary bodies and thalamic nuclei
    4. Temporo-parietal senile plaques and neurofibrillary tangles
    5. Cortical and subcortical nodules of primitive glial cells

30. Other symptoms that may develop as part of this illness include all of the following except:

    1. Chronic pancreatitis
    2. Splenic infarction
    3. Testicular atrophy
    4. Chronic insomnia
    5. Cardiomyopathy

31–33. An 8-year-old boy is referred for examination by his school teacher because of his restlessness in class. The teacher asks specifically that he be placed on methylphenidate. On examination, you find him to be shy, but cooperative. You note a recurrent nervous throat clearing and periodic shoulder shrugging.

31. Diagnostically he appears to be showing symptoms of:

    1. Lesch-Nyhan syndrome
    2. Separation anxiety disorder
    3. Autistic disorder
    4. Developmental articulation disorder
    5. Tourette's disorder

32. All of the following medications are used therapeutically in this syndrome except:

    1. D-penicillamine
    2. Clonazepam
    3. Haloperidol
    4. Clonidine
    5. Pimozide

33. All of the following statements about patients with this illness are correct except:

    1. Increased incidence of tic disorders in relatives
    2. Eventually will require institutional care
    3. Higher than expected incidence of attention deficit hyperactivity disorder
    4. Most often onset in grade school years
    5. Symptoms wax and wane over months

34–36. You have been treating a depressed, anxious, 47-year-old woman with phenelzine 15 mg three times a day. After four weeks of treatment, she is sleeping better, her appetite is improving, and her mood seems to be less despondent. One afternoon she calls for an appointment because she is feeling so bad. Quite suddenly she has developed palpitations, sweating, and a grinding headache.

34. You anticipate that she is suffering from:

    1. Acute anxiety attack
    2. Depressive somatization
    3. Hypertensive crisis
    4. Somatic delusions
    5. Hyperventilation syndrome

35. When you see her, you will ask especially about:

    1. Recent head injury
    2. Dietary intake
    3. Family conflicts or stresses
    4. Memory changes
    5. Recent infections

36. Her symptoms are produced by an excess of:

    1. Acetaldehyde
    2. Phenylalanine
    3. Protoporphyrins
    4. Serotonin
    5. Tyramine

37–40. A 26-year-old woman is brought in for examination because her husband has discovered that she is gorging food and vomiting. The patient confesses that, for over five years, she has secretly been binge eating and then inducing vomiting.

37. Physical examination of this patient is likely to show all of the following except:

    1. Abrasions on the back of her hands
    2. Erosion of the teeth
    3. Enlarged salivary glands
    4. Esophageal tears
    5. Fine lanugo hair on the limbs

38. The patient reported that she experiences "feeding frenzies." You anticipate she is likely to describe each of the following symptoms except:

    1. Bingeing on high-calorie, high-carbohydrate food
    2. Binges terminated due to abdominal pain
    3. Guilt and self-disgust after bingeing
    4. Persistent amenorrhea
    5. Laxative or diuretic abuse

39. Patients with these symptoms are more likely to exhibit which of the following?

1. Agoraphobia
2. Obsessive hand washing
3. Kleptomania
4. Fetishism
5. Compulsive masturbation

40. Several weeks later, she seeks an emergency appointment because of chest pain, shortness of breath, and generalized tiredness. You will ask particularly about:

    1. Ipecac use
    2. Laxative abuse
    3. Diuretic intake
    4. Vitamin overdose
    5. Thyroid abuse

41–43. A 33-year-old divorced secretary has a difficult day at work. Her supervisor gave her additional work to do and was most unsympathetic when she protested. Without further complaint, she finished her work, even though this made her late for her usual bus. When she arrived home, she found that her two children had not taken in the newspaper. Though they protested that they had been too busy preparing supper, she raged at them, swatted her son on the back when he argued, and sent them both to bed without food.

41. This woman's anger toward her family could be considered a manifestation of:

    1. Isolation
    2. Undoing
    3. Projection
    4. Dissociation
    5. Displacement

42. Upstairs, in his bedroom, her 10-year-old son, initially very angry, settles down to his homework and completes three days' study projects in a short period. His behavior could be described as a form of:

    1. Intellectualization
    2. Sublimation
    3. Repression
    4. Compensation
    5. Symbolization

43. The 8-year-old little girl had cowered in her chair when her mother was upset and, as quickly as she could, fled the room. Now on the telephone, she is giggling and telling her friend how funny the whole episode was. Her behavior is an example of:

    1. Denial
    2. Conversion
    3. Rationalization

4. Reaction formation
5. Identification

44–45. Nine months ago, a 33-year-old woman was reversing her car in her driveway when she accidently ran over and killed a 2-year-old neighbor child who had been playing under the car. Everyone, including the child's parents, agreed that the accident was not her fault, but she just cannot forget what happened. Repeatedly she finds herself remembering how the dead child looked when she found him. She keeps wondering if she could have heard him playing under the car. At night, she has difficulty sleeping and she has disturbing, fearful dreams. Since the accident, she has refused to drive. She does not eat well, is tired all of the time, and feels estranged from everyone, even her concerned husband.

44. The patient is manifesting symptoms of:

    1. Normal grief reaction
    2. Major depression
    3. Adjustment disorder with depression
    4. Panic disorder
    5. Post-traumatic stress disorder

45. All of the following statements about this syndrome are correct except:

    1. Sleep patterns resemble primary depression
    2. Group therapy often beneficial
    3. May have onset in elderly from events in the past
    4. Response of society to the situation appears to have no effect on the symptoms
    5. Can occur in very young children

DIRECTIONS: For questions 46–80, one or more of the alternatives given are correct. After you decide which choices are correct, record your answer according to the following:

(A) if alternatives 1, 2, and 3 only are correct.
(B) if alternatives 1 and 3 only are correct.
(C) if alternatives 2 and 4 only are correct.
(D) if alternative 4 only is correct.
(E) if all four alternatives are correct.

46–47. A 32-year-old woman is referred for treatment. She is sad, weeping, constantly praying. She states that she is the worst sinner in the world. She claims she hears Satan's voice telling her she is going to burn in Hell. In response to this voice, she has made repeated attempts to throw herself from a third-floor window.

46. To reduce her suicidal feelings and bring her symptoms under control quickly, which of the following treatments would be appropriate?

1. Electroconvulsive therapy
2. Lorazepam
3. Haloperidol
4. Doxepin

47. The family asks what side effect might be anticipated if electroconvulsive therapy were used and you advise them:

    1. Possible vertebral compression fractures
    2. Mild retrograde amnesia clearing after several months
    3. Transient hypertension
    4. Amenorrhea for several months

48-50. A 23-year-old male is brought to the emergency room for evaluation after he attacked a fellow worker without warning. The patient stated that this worker was spying on him, and he said that he could hear his colleagues whispering about him all the time, even at home.

48. Your possible diagnoses include:

    1. Cocaine intoxication
    2. Amphetamine-induced delusional disorder
    3. Paranoid schizophrenia
    4. Paranoid personality disorder

49. To help differentiate these diagnoses, which of the following would be useful?

    1. Electroencephalogram
    2. Amytal interview
    3. Minnesota Multiphasic Personality Inventory
    4. Blood and urine toxicology

50. The patient complains that insects are crawling across his arms and legs. No insects can be found on close inspection. His complaint is a manifestation of:

    1. Synesthesia
    2. Haptic hallucination
    3. Koro
    4. Formication

51-52. A 19-year-old male found lying in the park is brought for evaluation. He is mute, staring blankly, and, when his arms are raised, his limbs remain in that position.

51. In your evaluation of this patient, which of the following diagnoses are possible?

    1. Neuroleptic toxicity
    2. Schizophrenia
    3. Encephalitis
    4. Depression

52. Initial physical and laboratory examination are normal. Which of these procedures would be appropriate?

    1. Haloperidol intramuscularly
    2. Electroconvulsive therapy
    3. Diazepam intravenously
    4. Benztropine intramuscularly

53-55. A 53-year-old female, with a 30-year history of bipolar disorder, has been maintained satisfactorily on lithium for 12 years. She has taken her medications regularly, and has maintained a steady, responsible job. In recent months, she has complained of increasing depression, lethargy, and weight gain. She states she feels "old and worn out."

53. Immediate management for this patient should include:

    1. Discontinue lithium, start trazodone
    2. Discontinue lithium, initiate electroconvulsive therapy
    3. Continue present lithium dosage, add doxepin
    4. Request thyroid function studies

54. With this patient, which of the following tests is most sensitive in evaluation of thyroid function?

    1. T_3 level
    2. Antithyroid antibodies
    3. T_4 level
    4. Thyroid-stimulating hormone level

55. If hypothyroidism is confirmed, what would be the appropriate management of the patient's symptoms? The patient and family are fearful about any treatment change because, as they say, she has done so well on her lithium.

    1. Brief course of electroconvulsive therapy
    2. Start prednisone 20 mg twice daily
    3. Add methylphenidate 5 mg twice daily to present treatment
    4. Continue lithium, start thyroxine 0.05–0.2 mg per day

56-57. You are called to evaluate a 71-year-old male, two days after prostatic resection, because he is confused and restless. The patient complains that he cannot sleep because men are coming through his window at night.

56. As you evaluate this patient, which of the following conditions are diagnostically possible?

    1. Medication toxicity
    2. Electrolyte imbalance
    3. Urinary tract infection
    4. Diazepam withdrawal

57. While his condition is being evaluated, you could recommend which of the following management procedures?

1. Family member present around the clock
2. Night light in his room
3. Familiar photographs in his room
4. Remove monitor equipment from patient's view

58–59. An 82-year-old man consults you because of insomnia. He complains that he wakens at 3:00 or 4:00 AM, after going to bed at his usual 10:00 PM time. After he wakes up, he cannot go back to sleep, so usually he rises, reads a book, or watches television.

58. In your evaluation you will want to ask about:

1. Caffeine intake
2. Alcohol use
3. Affective state
4. Weight status

59. Your investigations show normal or negative findings. Accordingly you will recommend:

1. A program of daytime exercise so that he will be more tired at night
2. A small amount of alcohol regularly before going to bed
3. Low-dose benzodiazepine prior to going to bed
4. The patient does not need additional sleep at his age

60–61. A 72-year-old widow wishes to make a legally valid will. She seeks your advice about what evaluation procedures are necessary to ensure that she will be recognized as competent to make a will.

60. You advise her that the following need to be documented:

1. She knows how to read and write
2. She knows what she owns
3. She has no mental illness
4. She knows who her next of kin are

61. As you talk with her further, she confides in you that her daughter is poisoning her. She states that her water tastes "funny" and she thinks her daughter is putting LSD in the village water supply. Because of these beliefs, she refuses to leave this daughter, her only child, anything in her will. Which of the following statements are true about this patient?

1. She cannot be held legally responsible for her behavior
2. She should be committed to hospital based on her statements
3. You are legally obliged to notify the daughter of her mother's delusional feelings about her
4. She lacks testamentary capacity

62–64. A 4-year-old boy is scheduled to be hospitalized overnight, away from his farm home for a tonsillectomy.

62. In planning his management, you will recommend:

1. Parents stay with him overnight in hospital
2. Parents and doctor reassure him that he will not have any pain
3. Doctor demonstrates surgical procedures on a doll
4. Sedation should be started at home prior to admission to hospital

63. Following successful surgery, which of the following reactions might be anticipated?

1. Speaking baby talk
2. Thumb-sucking
3. Enuresis
4. Encopresis

64. About a year later, the little boy begins to experience nightmares of a monster coming into his bedroom. You advise the parents:

1. The little boy is manifesting post-traumatic stress disorder
2. A full neurological examination including electro-encephalography should be performed
3. Individual psychotherapy for the boy, parental therapy for the parents should be started
4. These symptoms are frequent at this age and usually transitory

65–68. You are asked to see a 3-year-old child because the parents are concerned that the youngster is not yet talking. He indicates what he wants by pointing or by noisy, wordless shout. The pediatrician, after examining him physically, has assured the parents that he will "grow out of it." As you watch the child in the waiting room, you note that he is a physically attractive little boy, sitting by himself and watching your grandfather clock across the room with interest. He appears rather placid, but when the chock chimes, he jumps up and down with excitement, waving his hands.

65. When a child of this age is not saying words, your differential diagnosis should include:

1. Deafness
2. Elective mutism
3. Infantile autism
4. Moderate mental retardation

66. Further examination shows no physical abnormalities. You note that the little boy always wants your examination room to be arranged the same way. Also he is fascinated by one of your windup toys with

which he spends most of his time. During the evaluation, you are likely to note:

1. Great difficulty separating from mother
2. Clinging and burrowing physically into mother
3. Open competitiveness with father
4. Easy unconcerned separation from mother

67. In your management of this youngster, which of the following are likely to be beneficial to the child during the next five years?

1. Moderate-dosage imipramine
2. Low-dosage haloperidol
3. Long-term supportive psychotherapy
4. Behavior modification training program

68. You advise the parents:

1. This syndrome typically occurs in middle or upper socioeconomic families
2. There is increased family incidence of this syndrome
3. These symptoms result from parental rejection or unpredictability
4. Most of these patients test at a retarded level

69–70. On the night after a championship football game, a 21-year-old out-of-town student is brought to the hospital emergency room in a confused state. He is sweating and tachycardiac. You note needle marks on his thighs and arms.

69. In your initial laboratory testing, you will want to include:

1. Cerebrospinal fluid protein
2. Urine toxicology
3. Urine porphyrins
4. Blood glucose

70. While you are awaiting test results, the patient is becoming more confused and disruptive. Your best initial management would be:

1. Intramuscular benztropine
2. Intravenous diazepam
3. Intramuscular haloperidol
4. Intravenous glucose

71–72. A middle-aged male is hospitalized after being found wandering the streets. He does not know his name, where he stays, or whether he has family. While he looks weather-beaten, physical and laboratory examinations, including electroencephalogram, show no major abnormalities. Toxic screen is negative. He is friendly, cooperative, and appears to be of average intelligence. He comes to your examination room from the recreational therapy department downstairs and, after your evaluation, returns unaided to his activities.

71. In your differential diagnosis, you are likely to include:

1. Alzheimer's disease
2. Psychogenic fugue
3. Conversion disorder
4. Malingering

72. To help clarify your diagnosis, you might use which of the following procedures?

1. Sodium amobarbital interview
2. Five to ten electroconvulsive therapy treatments
3. Hypnosis
4. Low-dose haloperidol

73–75. A 29-year-old school teacher consults you because she has been having recurrent "nervous attacks" for the past two years. These episodes, now occurring with increasing frequency, manifest with sudden, nearly overwhelming anxiety, sweating, tachycardia, difficulty breathing, weakness, and dizziness. In recent months, she has missed many days of work due to these attacks or fear that they might occur.

73. Her symptoms are liable to be induced by:

1. Cocaine abuse
2. 20 mg oral dose of yohimbine
3. Intravenous sodium lactate
4. Pheochromocytoma

74. Her symptoms can be treated on a long-term basis with:

1. Imipramine
2. Bupropion
3. Phenelzine
4. Diazepam

75. In your discussion of this syndrome, you advise the patient:

1. This syndrome is two to four times more common in women than in men
2. This syndrome is associated with high caffeine use
3. These symptoms are associated with temporal lobe seizures
4. These symptoms are commonly caused by hypoglycemia

76–78. A 32-year-old woman is hospitalized because she has stopped eating. She has been spending most of her time sitting silently in her bedroom staring at the wall. She states she is a wicked sinner, condemned by God. She believes that he has already died because of her sins, and now her intestines are rotting. Voices tell her that she should kill herself. She has obviously lost a great deal of weight, and she has started to refuse all fluids.

76. Useful procedures in the first week of treatment could include:

    1. Initiate electroconvulsive therapy
    2. Begin high-dose dozepin
    3. Start oral haloperidol
    4. Start long-range lithium

77. Your hospital management should include:

    1. Patient should be permitted to keep all her clothes and allowed to decorate her room with framed family photographs
    2. Continuous direct observation by staff including bathroom activities
    3. Family should be encouraged to take patient on short walks outside the hospital
    4. Careful physical examination including pelvic and rectal examination

78. The patient's husband asks whether electroconvulsive therapy would be beneficial. You advise him:

    1. Since the patient may have mitral stenosis, electroconvulsive therapy would be contraindicated
    2. A four to six week hospital stay would have to be planned to allow for the 15 to 20 treatments usually required
    3. Electroconvulsive therapy would limit his wife's artistic ability
    4. Electroconvulsive therapy is likely to cause several months' amenorrhea

79-80. You are asked to see a 58-year-old male because he complains of lack of energy, he has had frequent accidents at work, and he has become increasingly irritable. The patient is cooperative, verbal, and obviously concerned, but not depressed about the reported problems. His general health is good, though he is overweight. His wife reports that he is a restless sleeper.

79. You inquire specifically about:

    1. Bingeing and purging
    2. Sudden episodes of muscle paralysis
    3. Loss of sexual inhibitions
    4. Loud snoring during sleep

80. Appropriate management may include which of the following?

    1. ENT consultation
    2. Weight reduction
    3. Tracheostomy
    4. Low-dose short-acting benzodiazepine at bedtime

ANSWERS AND EXPLANATIONS

Case number 1–4

1. (3) *Anorexia nervosa* is an eating disorder, characterized by weight loss, leading to body weight of at least 15% below expected. Most of the weight loss is accomplished in secret. The syndrome is seen predominantly in females (90–95%), between the ages of 10 and 30 years and most commonly starting during early to late adolescence. Amenorrhea is common during menstrual years. (*CTP 1854–64. APA 755–59. Har 434–39.*)

2. (1) In addition to amenorrhea and weight loss, physical examination can reveal hypothermia (related to the severe weight loss), dependent edema, bradycardia, hypotension, and lanugo (appearance of neonatal-like hair). (*CTP 1854–64. APA 755–59. Har 434–39.*)

3. (2) Laboratory tests reveal the following: elevated base growth hormone levels, mild anemia, leukopenia and relative lymphocytosis, hypokalemic alkalosis (increased bicarbonate, hypochloremia, hypokalemia), and EKG changes (flattening or inverse of T waves, ST segment depression, and lengthening of QT interval). Some reports question whether cortisol production is actually increased as part of anorexia. (*CTP 1854–64. APA 755–59. APA 434–39.*)

4. (3) Eating disorders occur in all socioeconomic groups, but are more common in certain occupations (such as ballet). The risk of anorexia is higher (7%) for siblings of the patient, and children of parents who have problems of increased weight. There is a 2–5% risk of suicides in chronic anorexia nervosa patients. (*CTP 1854–64. APA 755–59. Har 434–39.*)

Case number 5–6

5. (1) Patients with factitious disorders, of which the best known is Munchausen's syndrome, are characterized by their pathological lying (pseudologia fantastica), patterns of extensive wandering from city to city and hospital to hospital, and their feigning of illness. These subjects will take anticoagulants to produce bleeding, contaminate urine with blood or feces, or even take insulin to produce hypoglycemia in order to receive medical care. (*APA 549–52. CTP 1136–40.*)

6. (2) Three main types of factitious disorders have been described as acute abdominal, hemorrhagic, and neurological, but there are many other forms involving every organ system. These patients are usually males, who show an unusual submissiveness and equanimity for hospital procedures and tests. If their tests are negative, they may become abusive, threaten litigation, and often sign out against medical advice. During evaluations they are likely to be evasive about details of prior treatments or investigations. (*APA 549–52. CTP 1136–40.*)

Case number 7–8

7. (3) Lithium may cause physical problems due to toxicity or sensitivity to the salt. Lithium blood levels should be obtained 12 hours after the last dose. A slow release form of lithium generally gives a constant 30% higher blood level over the day than the regular lithium salt form, which peaks and drops within hours. A rapid high rise in blood lithium can cause gastrointestinal problems, tremors, vision difficulties, and tinnitus. Too little sodium in food or from special diets and a decrease in body fluids from excessive sweating can lead to lithium toxicity (levels greater than 1.5 mEq/l). Treatment of an acute manic episode is likely to require lithium therapeutic blood levels of 0.8–1.2 mEq/liter, whereas maintenance blood levels are more likely to be 0.6–1.0 mEq/l. In some manic patients, blood levels as low as 0.4 Eq/l will maintain symptom relief. (*CTP 1655–62. APA 821–22. Har 502.*)

8. (1) Lithium is cleared primarily through renal excretion. Lithium is more likely to accumulate to toxic levels in the elderly due to age-related decreased renal functions. (*CTP 1659. APA 1137.*)

Case number 9–12

9. (3) Interviewing the child and family is the core skill of child psychiatry. The process of interviewing is essential to developing a therapeutic relationship and starts with the first contacts and initial meeting. (*APA 183. Har 614–15.*)

10. (4) Based on problems described and the psychiatric evaluation, the patient meets the criteria for a diagnosis of *attention deficit hyperactivity disorder* (ADHD) (DSM–III–R requires 8 of 14 criteria). The major symptoms for the ADHD diagnosis include motoric hyperactivity, impulsivity, inattention, and emotional liability. However, ADHD may be seen in association with other psychiatric disorders (dual diagnosis). (*CTP 1825–36. APA 652, 659–60.*)

11. (3) A variety of treatment modalities are useful, including environmental management, general education, and medications. Psychopharmacological treatment is nonspecific but usually involves psychostimulants or antidepressants (tricyclics or MAOIs). Benzodiazepines and barbiturates should be avoided, but diphenhydramine (Benadryl) and chloral hydrate can be used for sleep. (*APA 660–61.*)

12. (3) Approximately 10% of boys and 2% of girls of school age in the United States are reported to have ADHD. ADHD can be diagnosed at 36 months of age, but it is generally difficult to identify before age 5 due to

normal developmental hyperactivity. Most often these patients are not diagnosed until elementary school. ADHD is not a benign or self-limited childhood disorder, and many adults continue to show problems long after motoric hyperactivity is no longer prominent. It is reported that 25% of adults who had ADHD as children show antisocial personality disorders. ADHD is commonly seen with other childhood psychiatric disorders, particularly mood and conduct disorders. There is an overrepresentation of ADHD in patients with Tourette's disorder (20–60%) and obsessive compulsive disorder. (*CTP 1825–36. APA 652–64.*)

Case number 13–14
13. (5) *Acute intermittent porphyria* is an inborn error of metabolism, caused by an autosomal-dominant trait, more common in women, and most apt to appear after puberty and in the third or fourth decade of life. Recurrent abdominal pains or intense colic are common, often leading to unnecessary abdominal surgery. Symptoms of emotional instability are frequently present for long periods of time. Along with peripheral neuropathy and cranial nerve signs (ophthalmoplegia, facial palsy, dysphagia), these patients can show confusion, delirium, convulsions, and coma during acute attacks. (*CTP 1294–95.*)

14. (2) Since barbiturates, sulfonamides, grisofulvin, chloroquine, and certain steroids may precipitate or aggravate the attacks of acute porphyria, they must be avoided. During acute episodes, only symptomatic treatment is used as there are no specific treatments. Antipsychotic medications may be safely used to provide relief from pain and psychiatric symptoms. (*CTP 1294–95.*)

Case number 15–19
15. (3) *Neuroleptic malignant syndrome* (NMS), an increasingly diagnosed, potentially fatal reaction to antipsychotic medications, can occur at any time during treatment. The syndrome can present with severe akinetic and catatonic reactions, with an oral temperature of at least 37.5 C or 100.4 F (hyperpyrexia can go over 107 F), and increased respiratory rate and blood pressure. A milder bradykinesia and rigidity may precede the potentially catastrophic reaction. (*CTP 1624–25. APA 783–84. Har 495–96.*)

16. (1) NMS requires early recognition, immediate discontinuation of neuroleptic medications (do not give any other type of antipsychotic), intensive medical and nursing care (to cool patient, regulate blood pressure, and maintain renal output), and a search for infections or other treatable conditions. Antiparkinsonian drugs are usually not helpful and may actually contribute to a cerebral intoxication. (*CTP 1624–25. APA 783–84. Har 495–96.*)

17. (5) For the diagnostic criteria, see question 15. (*CTP 1624–25. APA 783–84. Har 495–96.*)

18. (1) Treatment is by the cautious use of the dopamine agonist bromocriptine mesylate (Parlodel), in oral or IM doses of 5–60 mg per day, or the muscle relaxant dantroline (Dantrium) 200 mg per day. Laboratory tests reveal increased WBC (greater than 15,000), blood creatinine phosphokinase (CPK, greater than 300 U/ml), liver enzymes, and myoglobin. These patients are likely to show profound muscle rigidity and rhabdomyolysis, which causes the release of creatine phosphokinase and myoglobin into the blood with resultant potentially fatal renal damage. (*CTP 1624–25. APA 783–84. Har 495–96.*)

19. (2) After an NMS incident, if neuroleptics are still indicated, they must be restarted slowly. The patient's response is not predictable. Some patients show an immediate NMS reaction when the same neuroleptic is restarted; others do not develop symptom recurrence. (*CTP 1624–25. APA 783–84. Har 495–96.*)

Case number 20–22
20. (3) The treatment of mania involves the use of immediate antipsychotic drugs, particularly the phenothiazines (chlorpromazine, haloperidol), as an adjunct to long-range lithium. Other drugs that are also useful in treating acute mania are carbamazepine, clonazepam, and sometimes valproic or IM lorazepam. Electroconvulsive therapy (ECT) is very effective in treating acute mania and may be most useful if there is a fear of complications from drug interactions. The standard treatment for mania is hospitalization, medications, and the use of restraints and seclusion if the patient is combative or violent. (*CTP 913–33. APA 430–33. Har 332–33, 583.*)

21. (3) The following procedures should be routinely performed before initiating lithium treatment: (1) pregnancy test for females of childbearing age, due to possible lithium teratogenicity; (2) EKG and blood pressure to assess cardiovascular status; (3) thyroid profile, T_3, T_4, and TSH, to rule out euthyroid goiter, or hypothyroidism; (4) genitourinary profile to include creatinine clearance to rule out glycosuria and nephrogenic diabetes insipidus; (5) complete blood count to evaluate leukocytosis. (*CTP 1660. APA 259–60.*)

22. (3) The most common problems associated with lithium use, especially when doses are increased rapidly, are nausea, vomiting, diarrhea, light-headedness, a resting tremor, polyuria, and weight gain. Other side effects seen with patients receiving lithium include EKG changes (flattening and inversion of T waves), hypotension, cardiac arrhythmias (rare), hypothyroidism, neutrophilia, acne vulgaris, and variable alopecia. (*CTP 1660–61. APA 822–27. Har 504–6.*)

Case number 23–25

23. **(4)** One of the variants of *Munchausen's syndrome*, called "Munchausen's by proxy," occurs when the parents present their child with a fabricated illness. Mothers of these children are more likely to have had nursing training and a history of a factitious illness themselves. (*CTP 1137–38. APA 551.*)

24. **(2)** Mothers refuse to leave the hospital and usually appear very solicitous about the child. Parents of these children may show a lack of appropriate concern about the child's illness. In addition, the children may improve clinically or may not show signs and symptoms of the illness in the parent's absence. (*CTP 1137–38. APA 551.*)

25. **(2)** The disorder in the parent who produces the child's symptoms seems to be related to personality and character trait difficulties, such as depressive-masochistic, borderline, psychopathic and antisocial personality disorders. The parent usually has average or above average intelligence, an absence of formal thought disorder, and often a poor sense of personal and sexual identity. (*CTP 1137–38.*)

Case number 26–30

26. **(3)** An *alcohol withdrawal syndrome* can begin within several hours of stopping or reducing prolonged heavy drinking. It starts with the development of coarse tremors of the hands, tongue, and eyelids and is likely to occur with at least one of the following symptoms: nausea or vomiting; malaise or weakness; autonomic hypersensitivity; anxiety, depressed mood, or irritability; transient hallucinations or illusions; headaches. (*CTP 201–2, 686–98. APA 316.*)

27. **(4)** Treatment of alcohol withdrawal involves the aggressive use of vitamin B$_{12}$, folic acid (1 mg), and thiamine (100 mg IM), plus high doses of medications consisting mainly of the benzodiazepines, or magnesium sulfate and phenobarbital if benzodiazepines are contraindicated. Other drugs to consider are the phenothiazines, if psychosis is present, chloral hydrate for sleep, and clonidine or propranolol if increased blood pressure or pulse rate is a problem. The routine use of phenytoin (Dilantin) to prevent seizures is not necessary. Intravenous (IV) electrolytes and dextrose and water may be needed, but overhydration is likely in these patients rather than dehydration. (*CTP 1434. APA 324–25. Har 709.*)

28. **(1)** *Wernicke-Korsakoff syndrome* is an encephalopathy presenting with truncal ataxia, ophthalmoplegia, and mental confusion. The etiology is believed to be thiamine deficiency. The syndrome may not improve despite abstinence from alcohol and maintenance on thiamine therapy. (*CTP 639. APA 293, 323. Har 363.*)

29. **(3)** On postmortem examination, there is likely to be hemorrhage and sclerosis of both the hypothalamic mammillary bodies and nuclei of the thalamus as well as less specific and more diffuse lesions of the brainstem, cerebellum, and limbic system. (*CTP 639. APA 293, 323. Har 363.*)

30. **(2)** *Korsakoff's psychosis* and *alcoholic dementia* can be seen in about 2% of patients with alcohol dependency. Patients with primary alcoholism have a death rate three times greater than their nonalcoholic age group as well as higher rates of suicide and violent crimes. Medical complications are common, including gastritis, ulcers, pancreatitis, esophageal varices, hypoglycemia, anemia, cardiomyopathy, peripheral neuropathy, sexual dysfunctions, liver disease, cancer, fetal alcohol syndrome, subdural hematoma, seizures, and chronic pulmonary infections (especially tuberculosis). *CTP 639. APA 317. Har 710.*)

Case number 31–33

31. **(5)** Tic disorders are classified into transient tics (usually motor), chronic tics, and Tourette's disorder. 5–24% of school age children have histories of tics. Tourette's disorder presents with a characteristic triad (in about one-third of cases) of:

    1. motor tics, in the neck, face and sometimes lower limbs
    2. vocal tics, ranging from throat clearing to snorting, hissing, barking, swearing, or profanity (coprolalia)
    3. obsessive compulsive symptomatology, which includes recurring thoughts, repetitive touching, collecting, orderliness, or self-mutilation (*CTP 1865. APA 684. Har 123.*)

32. **(1)** Treatment of tics is by behavioral techniques, medications such as minor tranquilizers, low doses of major neuroleptics, and psychosocial interventions. The mainstay of treatment of Tourette's disorder is the use of dopamine-blocking agents. With Tourette's disorder, about 60–80% of patients respond to low doses (0.5–5 mg/day) of haloperidol, but other neuroleptics can be used. Pimozide may be useful and clonidine helps in about one-half of cases; stimulants and certain antidepressants may exacerbate existing tics or produce new tics. (*CTP 1865. APA 686–88.*)

33. **(2)** The onset of Tourette's disorder is typically from 2 to 13 years (though some reports state 6–20 years), and the syndrome is more common in males. It is a lifelong disease showing a characteristic waxing and waning in frequency and severity. Genetic, biological, and psychosocial factors appear operative in all tic disorders. Two-thirds of the relatives of Tourette's disorder patients have tics; there is an increased incidence in obsessive compulsive disorders in family members and a higher incidence in monozygotic than dizygotic twins. There ap-

pears to be a genetic link among Tourette's disorder, chronic tics, obsessive compulsive disorders, and ADHD. (*APA 687.*)

Case number 34–36

34. (3) (*CTP 1651–52. APA 802–3. Har 519.*)

35. (2)(Reference—see Question 34.)

36. (5) Phenelzine sulfate (Nardil), an MAO inhibitor, lacks anticholinergic activity, but produces autonomic side effects such as dry mouth and dysfunction of bowel and bladder. Sexual dysfunctions, orthostatic hypotension, hepatotoxic reactions, agitation, insomnia, confusion, and toxic psychosis can occur with increasing dosage. If MAOIs are taken with certain foods, medications, or beverages containing sympathomimetic amines, such as tyramine (a fermentation product), an acute hypertensive crisis can be produced, with the risk of intracranial bleeding and cardiovascular collapse. (Reference—see Question 34.)

Case number 37–40

37. (5) In *bulimia nervosa,* an eating disorder, problems develop as a result of the bingeing and purging. These patients may show dental enamel erosions, abrasions and scars on knuckles (from inducing vomiting, "Russell's sign"), enlarged parotid glands, amenorrhea, hypokalemia, and esophagitis with tears. If a bulimic patient uses ipecac chronically, cardiomyopathy can develop. (See question 40.) (*CTP 1854–64. APA 760–61. Har 436.*)

38. (4) Bulimics binge on high caloric foods and develop abdominal pains, which may end the bingeing episode. They tend to abuse laxatives in an attempt to control weight. Many manifest symptoms of anxiety, depression, and compulsive behavior. (*CTP 1854–64. APA 760–61. Har 436.*)

39. (3) Associated with this disorder are impulsive stealing (especially food, clothing, jewelry), chemical dependency (especially alcohol), and abuse of amphetamines. (*CTP 1854–64. APA 760.*)

40. (1) Chronic ipecac abuse can produce a cardiomyopathy. Precordial pain, dyspnea, hypotension, tachycardia, and EKG abnormalities should alert the physician to the possibility of ipecac intoxication. (*APA 761.*)

Case number 41–43

41. (5) *Displacement* is the defense mechanism used when emotions, ideas, and wishes are transferred from their original less acceptable object to a more acceptable substitute. Defenses are unconscious, manage instincts and affects, and can be adaptive as well as pathological. (*CTP 375–76. APA 135–38, 1249. Har 201–3, 217–22.*)

42. (2) *Sublimation* is the defense used when unacceptable instinctual drives are diverted into personally and socially acceptable channels. (*CTP 375. APA 1268. Har 222.*)

43. (4) *Reaction formation* is a defense mechanism used when the subject manifests affects, ideas, attitudes, and behaviors that are opposite to the actual but unacceptable feelings. (*CTP 376. APA 1268. Har 220.*)

Case number 44–45

44. (5) *Post-traumatic stress disorder* (PTSD) has three major features that are central to the disorder: (1) episodic, involuntary, and vividly intrusive recollections, daydreams, or nightmares of the trauma; (2) excessive autonomic arousal such as chronic anxiety, hypervigilance, sleeplessness, irritability, and sudden outbursts of violent or destructive behavior; and (3) psychic numbing to emotions of intimacy, tenderness, and sexual interest, emotional detachment from people, and loss of interest in places and activities. (*CTP 1000–1008. Har 245. APA 479.*)

45. (3) Crisis intervention after the traumatic event appears to reduce immediate distress and possibly prevent chronic or delayed responses. Time-limited psychotherapy, group and family therapy, and the use of social support systems are useful treatment procedures. Antidepressant medication may be helpful, especially when both a PTSD and a major affective disorder may coexist. Symptoms can appear acutely (one week) after the stress or be delayed until months or even years later (after 30 years or longer), and can occur at any age (as in adults who were child victims of abuse or burns). (*CTP 1000–1008. APA 485, 483. Har 245.*)

Case number 46–47

46. (B) Electroconvulsive therapy should be considered as the initial treatment if the patient is severely depressed, especially if delusional, and at a high risk for suicide. In an emergency situation, rapid neuroleptization by the use of high-potency antipsychotics (particularly oral or parental haloperidol) gives speedy resolution of symptoms. (*APA 387, 432. Har 583–84.*)

47. (E) The most common side effects of electroconvulsive therapy are headaches, muscle aches, and cardiovascular changes (transient fluctuations in BP during and shortly after treatments). Cognitive and memory problems are less with unilateral placement of electrodes on the nondominant hemisphere (i.e., right handed on right side). The use of general anesthesia poses the biggest risk. Amenorrhea, a recognized side effect of ECT, is not usually mentioned in current textbooks. Brainstem herniation can occur during ECT if the patient has a space occupying cerebral lesion. Monoamine oxidase inhibitors potentiate barbiturate anesthesia and increase the hypertensive response seen during ECT. (*APA 838–40. CTP 1670–78. Har 582–83.*)

Case number 48–50

48. **(A)** Paranoid delusions and hallucination can be symptomatic of many medical and neurological disorders:

    1) neurological disorders—seizures, Parkinson's, Huntington's, dementias (Alzheimer's, Pick's)
    2) vitamin deficiency states
    3) drug induced—cocaine, phencyclidine, THC, LSD, mescaline, amphetamines, anticholinergics, disulfiram
    4) systemic—porphyria, uremia, and hypoglycemia

    Paranoid personality disorder does not have the psychotic delusional or hallucinatory content seen in schizophrenia or the cognitive changes noted as part of organic mental disorders. (*CTP 671. APA 337–43, 630. Har 303.*)

49. **(D)** Part of the evaluation should include a toxicology screen and a routine blood and urine laboratory series, neuropsychological tests for cognitive impairment (i.e., Bender Gestalt, Wechsler Memory Scale), EEG, or possibly a CAT scan, or MRI. (*CTP 671.*)

50. **(C)** *Formication* is a delusional sensation that insects are crawling under the skin and occurs commonly in delirium tremens and cocainism ("cocaine bugs").

    A *haptic* (tactile) *hallucination* is the false perception of touch or surface sensation when no stimulus is present. It occurs principally in toxic states and with certain addictions.

    Synesthesia is a sensation or hallucination in one sensory modality caused by another sensation modality (e.g., auditory stimuli trigger a visual image: seeing sounds).

    Koro is an acute anxiety reaction characterized by patient's fear that the penis is shrinking, may disappear into his abdomen, and he may die.

    Kuru is a progressive dementia accompanied by extrapyramidal signs and found when brains infected with slow virus are eaten. (*Har 40. APA 189. CTP 671.*)

Case number 51–52

51. **(E)** *Catatonia* is abnormal posturing with motor, sensory, and verbal symptoms, and includes verbigeration, mutism, negativism, stereotyped movements, waxy flexibility, and decreased sensitivity to pain.

    Cerea flexibilitas, "waxy flexibility," is present when a patient's arm or leg remains fixed in a placed position. Either symptom can be seen in catatonic schizophrenia, affective and organic mental disorders, viral encephalitis, frontal lobe tumors, metabolic disorders (e.g., acute intermittent porphyria), toxic reactions, or as drug-in-

duced extrapyramidal side effects of antipsychotics. (*APA 365, 371–72. Har 37.*)

52. **(D)** To provide rapid treatment, use the two parental (IM and IV) forms of anticholinergic drugs, benztropine mesylate (Cogentin) or diphenhydramine (Benadryl). Trihexyphenidyl (Artane), or amantadine (Symmetrel) by oral route can also be used. (*APA 779–80. Har 494.*)

Case number 53–55

53. **(D)** About 20% of patients on lithium develop hypothyroidism: hypothyroidism occurs more frequently with female patients, patients with thyroid antibodies, or in patients with exaggerated TSH response to TRH. (*CTP 1661–62. APA 824–25. Har 504–6.*)

54. **(C)** Before the initiation of lithium treatment, initial laboratory tests should include a thyroid profile with T_3RU, T_4RIA, T_4I, and TSH. An abnormal TSH and presence of antithyroid antibodies are the most sensitive tests for detecting subclinical hypothyroidism. (*APA 822–25. Har 506.*)

55. **(D)** If the patient needs to be maintained on lithium, supplemental exogenous thyroxin, 0.05–0.2 mg/day, should be given as this usually leads to the regression of the goiter. Otherwise, it may be necessary to discontinue lithium and use another antimanic medication. (*CTP 1661–62. APA 824. Har 506.*)

Case number 56–57

56. **(E)** The recent onset of a sudden change in thinking and behavior in a patient with recognized medical disease and no previous psychiatric history suggests delirium (acute confusional state) rather than a functional psychosis. Delirium is usually secondary to a pathological process outside the CNS, but may be due to a primary disease of the brain. The most common causes are derangements of normal body metabolism (i.e., metabolic imbalance) leading to toxins (e.g., hypoxia, hypoglycemia, vitamin B_1 deficiency), or from endocrine disorders, infections, postoperative states, drug intoxications and withdrawal states, and neurological diseases (e.g., following seizures, head trauma). (*CTP 624–29. APA 282–84. Har 362–65.*)

57. **(A)** The treatment of underlying illness primarily involves correction of fluids or electrolyte imbalances, treatment of infections, and drug withdrawal procedures. General nursing measures include keeping the room well lighted and avoiding loud noises and any unnecessary movements. The patient should not be immediately transferred to a psychiatric unit. The strange surroundings of the hospital room should be made more familiar by (1) having relatives bring items from home (e.g., family picture, clock, home cooked meals); (2) limiting the number of changes in the patient's nurses,

physicians; (3) restricting visitors to those close to patient; (4) decreasing time away from the ward for procedures; and (5) keeping the TV tuned in to regularly listened to programs. (*CTP 624–29. APA 305. Har 365–66.*)

Case number 58–59

58. **(E)** The elderly are likely to complain of insomnia or sleeplessness. A healthy older person typically lies awake for one-fifth of the night, and has more frequent awakenings. Older subjects experience an increase in sleep disordered breathing and nocturnal myoclonus. Excessive liquids at night, especially caffeinated beverages and alcohol (requiring going to the bathroom), in addition to tobacco use, changes in weight and resultant hunger, and catnaps during the daytime must be ruled out. Other disorders such as delirium, affective disorders, and psychotic reactions must be considered. (*CTP 86–90. APA 740–43. Har 666.*)

59. **(D)** If all findings are normal, reassuring the patient that the changes are part of the aging process is appropriate and can be therapeutic. (*CTP 86–90. APA 740–43. Har 666.*)

Case number 60–61

60. **(C)** Competency and incompetency are always specific and time-dependent variables, and refer to the ability to perform a *specific* task (i.e., make a will, marry, divorce) rather than being global or general. Competence involves the patient's ability to understand the nature and consequence of her actions in the particular situation at issue. Competency to make a will is called testamentary capacity and requires answers to the following questions. Is she aware that she is signing a will? Is she able to assess the quantity and quality of her property? Is she able to understand who her heirs are? Is she under the undue influence of any party to the process? Further, she must appreciate the relations of these facts to one another, and have sufficient mind and memory to understand all the facts. (*CTP 2114. APA 1069–70. Har 820–21.*)

61. **(D)** Competency is a legal concept. Everyone is assumed to be competent in all respects unless determined otherwise by due legal process. Since there are elements of her mental state that disqualify her from meeting the cognitive capacity test, she lacks testamentary capacity. (*Har 820–21.*)

Case number 62–64

62. **(B)** Some degree of separation anxiety is a normal developmental phenomenon, especially during the first 18–30 months. Separation anxiety disorder is not typically observed before 4 years of age. The family can help the child by providing a consistent, supportive, caring environment. (*CTP 1970–74. APA 675.*)

63. **(E)** Regression is a common normal reaction after medical and surgical hospitalization and is stress related. Functional enuresis may be related to stress, trauma, hospitalization, or developmental crisis. Onset of stuttering during latency is often stress related and runs a benign course. Some reports state that stress-related factors appear causative in one-half of cases of secondary encopresis. (*Har 598. APA 689, 691, 693.*)

64. **(D)** Multiple phobias, especially of animals and darkness, are common in preschool children, with fear of dark, storms, heights seen transiently in one-half of 6–12-year-olds. (*CTP 1970–74. APA 672.*)

Case number 65–68

65. **(B)** *Infantile autism* is a major subclass of pervasive developmental disorder (PDD). Symptoms of infantile autism include: (1) limited capacity for reciprocal social interaction (i.e., aloofness, social detachment); (2) impaired ability to communicate; (3) restricted repertoire of activities and interests; and (4) onset during infancy or early childhood.

The ability to use words communicatively should normally begin by 18 months of age, with the use of phrases by 2½–3 years of age. Children with elective mutism usually have normal speech development, but do not speak in one or several major environments in which they live. Differential diagnosis in PDD should include congenital deafness, defects in hearing acuity, developmental expressive and receptive language disorders, and neurological problems (aphasia). (*CTP 1779–82. APA 694. Har 619.*)

66. **(D)** Children with autistic disorder show low social interactiveness, a seemingly indifference to human warmth, and little imitation or sharing. Initially they avoid social contact, but eventually they can come to enjoy and seek interpersonal experiences. They pursue narrow interests in activity, may become attached to unusual objects and distressed over any changes in environment. (*CTP 1779–82. APA 712–13.*)

67. **(C)** Treatment uses a multimodal approach over a long period of time and may include special education, psychotropic medications, behavior therapy, parental guidance, and residential treatment. Medications may consist of low doses of nonsedating neuroleptics, such as haloperidol, 2–10 mg per day, or psychostimulants, such as fenfluramine, if there is a concurrent ADHD. The opiate receptor blocking agents, such as naltrexone, may have a helpful effect according to some reports by improving social and affective responsiveness, and reducing stereotyped motor and self-injurious behavior. (*CTP 1779. APA 716.*)

68. **(C)** Infantile autism occurs across all socioeconomic levels. A higher concordance occurs in monozygotic twins

(36%) compared with no concordance with dizygotic twins. Commonly associated problems are mental retardation (only 2–15% achieve nonretarded level of cognitive and adaptive functioning) and seizure disorders (35–50% by age 20). (*CTP 1785–86. APA 714–15.*)

Case number 69–70

69. **(C)** Hypoglycemia symptoms usually occur when blood glucose level drops or remains below 50 mg/dl (women 40 mg/dl). Patients may appear as having an anxiety or depressive disorder and show nervousness, tremor, agitation, confusion, sweating, dizziness, weakness, fatigue, hunger, and sweating during a hypoglycemia episode. If possible, blood glucose levels should be drawn when the patient is maximally symptomatic. (*APA 522–23.*)

70. **(D)** Intravenous glucose will promptly relieve acute symptoms of hypoglycemia. (*APA 523.*)

Case number 71–72

71. **(C)** *Fugue state* (psychogenic fugue) manifests by a sudden state of identity change during which the individual gives up customary habits and lifestyle, wanders far from home, and sets up a new life as a seemingly different person. The patient may suddenly recover the original identity after a period of weeks or months and be mystified and distressed to be in a strange place with strange people. There is total amnesia for all the time of the fugue. A malingerer may develop apparent amnesia because of a vested interest in failing to recall a certain event to avoid some responsibility or commitment. In differentiating psychogenic amnesia from psychogenic fugue, the former does not involve purposeful travel or a new identity. (*CTP 1034–36. APA 569. Har 100, 247.*)

72. **(B)** The distinction between genuine and feigned amnesia may be difficult. Hypnosis and sodium amobarbital ("Amytal") interviews may be of value, but some individuals continue to malinger under these procedures. (*CTP 1034–35. APA 565.*)

Case number 73–75

73. **(E)** *Anxiety disorder*. may have symptoms similar to many physical illnesses such as hyperthyroidism, hypothyroidism, hyperparathyroidism, hypoglycemia, pheochromocytoma, Meniere's disease, mitral valve prolapse, cardiac arrhythmias, drug reactions (cocaine, yohimbine, isoproterenol), and inhalation of carbon dioxide (CO_2). (*CTP 965–69. APA 448–50, 454. Har 237.*)

74. **(B)** Treatment of severe anxiety or panic disorder is primarily by tricyclic (imipramine) or MAOI (phenelzine) antidepressants. Other drugs that can be used are the benzodiazepine derivatives, alprazolam and clonazepam, the nonbenzodiazepine antianxiety agent busiprone, and the alpha and beta adrenergic blocking drugs propranolol and clonidine. (*APA 457. Har 238, 536. CTP 970–72.*)

75. **(A)** Panic disorder without agoraphobia occurs equally in males and females, but panic disorder with agoraphobia is seen in females two times more often than in males. The mean age of onset is age 25. Excessive caffeine intake may exacerbate the symptoms of panic, but hypoglycemia is rarely the cause. (*CTP 960–69.*)

Case number 76–78

76. **(B)** Antipsychotic medications are used in treating acute psychotic episodes, in maintaining remission of schizophrenia, and in amelioration of psychotic symptoms from a variety of causes that include affective disorders with psychotic features, drug or medication toxicities (e.g., steroid psychosis), brain disorders (e.g., Huntington's disease or post-head injury), and acute manic symptoms.

The principal indications for electroconvulsive therapy (ECT) are severe or delusional depression especially when symptoms are intense, prolonged, with profound alterations in vegetative functioning, suicidal activity, and psychomotor retardation, and catatonia or acute mania. (*CTP 1673–75. APA 774, 837. Har 583.*)

77. **(C)** When a patient shows delusional suicidal ideation, constant observation is required. Contraindications or reasons for caution for ECT would be significant cardiovascular problems, particularly hypertension, cerebral mass (neoplasms), degenerative diseases of the spine or other bones, and preexisting MAOI treatment. Therefore, a pre-ECT evaluation should consist of a complete medical and neurological examination, CBC, blood chemistries, urinalysis, and X-rays of lumbo-sacral region and chest. (*CTP 1673–75. APA 838. Har 584.*)

78. **(D)** Common side effects are headaches, muscle aches, and memory impairment, which is generally a retrograde amnesia. The amnesia usually clears within six months after treatments. (*CTP 1661–68. APA 840. Har 582–83.*)

Case number 79–80

79. **(D)** The essential feature of a sleep disorder is excessive daytime sleepiness or sleep attacks that are severe enough to impair the patient's social or occupational functioning. Obstructive sleep apnea syndrome, upper airway occlusion to airflow, is usually seen in middle-aged, overweight, and hypertensive men. Bed partners typically complain of the patient's loud snoring. (*CTP 1115. APA 745–46.*)

80. **(A)** A polysomnograph evaluation helps in formulating the specific type of sleep problem and treatment plan. An ENT evaluation is essential to determine if tongue retaining devices, modified tracheotomy, or continuous positive airway pressure is indicated. A treatment program to reduce weight and hypertension is required. (*APA 746. Har 153, 166.*)

11

MOCK EXAMINATION

DIRECTIONS: Select the best answer from the alternatives offered in questions 1 through 41.

1. All of the following statements about disulfiram treatment with alcoholics are correct except:

   1. Blocks metabolism of acetaldehyde
   2. May induce depression
   3. Liable to have toxic reaction with cough syrups
   4. Helpful in preventing deterioration in alcoholic dementia
   5. Can cause dangerous hypotension

2. According to Holmes and Rahe, which of the following events causes the most life stress?

   1. Birth of first child
   2. Marriage
   3. Death of parent
   4. Death of spouse
   5. Imprisonment

3. Subtracting 7 from 100 in a serial fashion tests primarily:

   1. Memory
   2. Mathematical ability
   3. Attention
   4. Orientation
   5. Abstract thinking

4. According to Heinz Kohut, narcissistic personality disorders are caused by:

   1. Disruption in evolution of empathically based self-objects
   2. Fixation at infantile autoerotic phase
   3. Persistence of paranoid schizoid position
   4. Disturbance of rapprochement phase
   5. Regression to oral phase of development

5. Effective treatment for neuroleptic induced akathisia would be which of the following?

   1. L-tryptophan
   2. Valproic acid
   3. Imipramine
   4. Methyldopa
   5. Propranolol

6. The inability to recognize one's own emotional feelings and to describe them in words is called:

   1. Extinction
   2. Alexithymia
   3. Hypesthesia
   4. Overcompensation
   5. Dysarthria

7. When stimulants are used to treat attention deficit hyperactivity disorder, all of the following statements are correct except:

   1. Decreased impulsivity
   2. Rebound effects when medication stopped
   3. Improved attention
   4. Improved reading skills in dyslexia
   5. May precipitate tic disorder

8. In chronic alcoholics, thiamine deficiency will produce all of the following symptoms except:

   1. Truncal ataxia
   2. Nystagmus
   3. 6th cranial nerve paralysis
   4. Seizures
   5. Amnesia

9. The earliest sign of puberty in the normally developing girl is:

   1. Onset of menses
   2. Rapidly increasing height
   3. Appearance of axillary hair
   4. Breast bud development
   5. Appearance of pubic hair

10. All of the following statements about homosexual rape are correct except:

    1. Victim often fears becoming homosexual
    2. Victim likely to experience sexual dysfunction
    3. Victim prone to blame himself
    4. Typically full recovery within a year
    5. Dynamics of rape similar to those in heterosexual rape

11. In working with patients, Kohut places much emphasis on:

    1. Resistances
    2. Real relationship
    3. Intuition

4. Countertransference
5. Empathy

12. All of the following statements about postpartum psychoses are correct except:

1. Recurrence over 50% in future pregnancies
2. Most patients with first episode postpartum psychoses have prior psychiatric history
3. Highest incidence in first month postpartum
4. Not related to obstetrical complications
5. Major risk of suicide or infanticide

13. A supervisor is obligated to ensure that a resident performs at the standard of the psychiatric profession. This obligation is defined by the legal doctrine:

1. Parens patriae
2. Mens rea
3. Respondeat superior
4. Res ipsa loquitur
5. Pro bono publico

14. In a hotly contested election, one of the candidates has made very definite and very opinionated statements. On a radio talk show about child development, the psychiatrist is asked to comment on the psychiatric status of this candidate. The appropriate response would be:

1. Refuse to talk about the candidate personally, but discuss the theoretical aspects of his comments
2. Refuse to answer the question, stating it would be unethical to do so
3. Defer the question to a later planned specific discussion about the election
4. Express your opinion, but clearly indicate that it is based only on what you have heard
5. Give as accurate a response as possible, but only in comparison with other candidates

15. Frequency at a point in time is:

1. Concordance rate
2. Specificity rate
3. Incidence rate
4. Prevalence rate
5. Relative risk

16. All of the following statements about benzodiazepines are correct except:

1. Abrupt withdrawal after chronic use may cause seizures
2. Intramuscular diazepam useful in anesthetic induction
3. Alcohol use may precipitate overdose
4. Withdrawal symptoms may mimic reemergence of original anxiety
5. Severity of withdrawal symptoms proportional to dose taken

17. All of the following statements about Tourette's disorder are correct except:

1. Onset usually preadolescent
2. Symptoms wax and wane
3. Coprolalia occurs in most cases
4. Relatives of affected females more often affected than relatives of male Tourette patients
5. Does not result in intellectual deterioration

18. Which of the following statements is applicable to reactive attachment disorder?

1. Reaction to loss of nurturing person in second six months of life
2. Described by Spitz as "anaclitic depression"
3. Manifested by separation anxiety
4. Caused by grossly neglectful and inadequate caregiving
5. Similar to adult mourning

19. All of the following statements about Down's syndrome are correct except:

1. Usually mild-to-moderate retardation
2. Difficult to place for adoption
3. Increased risk of seizure disorder
4. Muscular hypotonia
5. Chronic otis media common

20. All of the following statements about pathological gambling are correct except:

1. Generally starts during adolescence
2. Frequently associated with bulimia nervosa
3. Liable to have withdrawal irritability and restlessness
4. Treatment similar to that for alcoholism
5. Parents often pathological gamblers

21. Which of the following would be an example of primary prevention?

1. Suicide hotline
2. Sheltered workshops
3. Improved mental health insurance coverage
4. AIDS education in high school
5. Development of psychiatry emergency program

22. All of the following statements about imipramine are correct except:

1. May cause disabling orthostatic hypotension at therapeutic levels
2. Therapeutically contraindicated with ventricular arrhythmias
3. Increased risk of heart block at therapeutic levels
4. Overdose fatality usually due to cardiac rhythm disturbances
5. Most overdose deaths occur in first 24 hours after overdose

23. All of the following statements about psychiatrist-patient privileged communication are correct except:

1. Waived when patient suing the doctor
2. Waived when patient claims emotional harm in a legal suit
3. Waived in patient's best interest on physician's decision
4. Waived on patient's decision or demand
5. Waived in military court cases

24. All of the following statements about transference are correct except:

1. Present in all forms of psychotherapy
2. Revival of past relationship feelings
3. Analysis of transference is major technique of psychoanalysis
4. Positive transference may be expression of resistance
5. Refers to the therapist-patient working collaboration

25. Correct statements about suicide in the United States include all of the following except:

1. Highest rate in white males
2. Highest rate in adolescents and young adults
3. High rate in alcoholics
4. High risk with previous suicide attempt
5. High risk in heroin addicts

26. All of the following statements about impotence are correct except:

1. Most common organic cause is diabetes mellitus
2. Frequent side effect of trazodone
3. Cause for noncompliance with neuroleptics
4. Common side effect of antihypertensive medications
5. May be manifestation of cocaine abuse

27. All of the following statements about the psychiatrist as an expert witness are correct except:

1. Required to be board certified
2. Resident in training may be an expert witness
3. Pretrial consultation with attorney is helpful
4. Cannot be obliged to give "yes" or "no" answers
5. May be expected to comment on hearsay evidence

28. All of the following statements about placebo are correct except:

1. Pain relief in 35–40% of patients
2. Placebo effect does not differentiate whether pain is organically based
3. Placebo does not have side effects
4. Anxiety level predicts placebo response
5. Naloxone blocks analgesic effect of placebo

29. All of the following statements apply to the sleep apnea syndrome except:

1. Frequent impaired work performance
2. Typically obese males
3. Loud snoring disturbs sleeping partner
4. Frequent hypnagogic hallucinations
5. May require tracheostomy

30. "My mind just went blank" is an example of:

1. Thought insertion
2. Dissociation
3. Suppression
4. Blocking
5. Isolation

31. All of the following statements about elective mutism are correct except:

1. Refusal to speak in specific social situations
2. Frequently communicate nonverbally
3. Onset usually in preschool years
4. Behavior patterns often similar to 2-year-old child
5. Predominantly male

32. A small toy is placed inside a box in sight of an 18-month-old child. The child goes to the box, opens it, and retrieves the toy. According to Piaget, the child has achieved:

1. Conservation of quantity
2. Conservation of substance
3. Object constancy
4. Object permanence
5. Object relations

33. All of the following statements about bipolar disorder are correct except:

1. Bout of illness tends to last less than six months
2. Shorter episodes of illness than unipolar
3. Cycles tend to lengthen with age
4. Cycles tend to be shorter than unipolar
5. Recurrent mania without depression is classified as bipolar

34. Patients with bulimia are liable to show which of the following symptoms?

1. Frotteurism
2. Tic disorder
3. Kleptomania
4. Dyslexia
5. Sleep terror disorder

35. In the United States, most patients with mental disorders receive care from:

1. Psychiatrists and social workers in mental health centers
2. Primary care physicians in private offices

3. Mental health professionals in private offices
4. Physicians and nurses in state mental hospitals
5. Nonmedical personnel in nonmedical settings

36. According to Erik Erikson, the developmental task in normal middle age is concerned with:

1. Integrity
2. Intimacy
3. Industry
4. Generativity
5. Isolation

37. The Ganser syndrome is an example of:

1. Pseudocyesis
2. Pseudologica fantastica
3. Paraphrenia
4. Psychasthenia
5. Pseudodementia

38. The kappa statistic measures:

1. Degree of agreement beyond chance
2. Capacity of testing instrument to give consistent results
3. Comparison of sample with standard population
4. Deviation around the mean
5. Ability of a test to measure what it is supposed to measure

39. Opioid overdose is treated with:

1. Clonidine
2. Methadone
3. Naloxone
4. Diazepam
5. Propranolol

40. You are asked to evaluate a 5-year-old boy who, following the birth of a brother, began sucking his thumb and wetting his bed at night. You advise the parents that these symptoms are most likely manifestations of:

1. Repression
2. Castration anxiety
3. Regression
4. Reaction formation
5. Autism

41. Which of the following statements about functional enuresis is correct?

1. Frequently caused by harsh training
2. More likely to have smaller than average bladder capacity
3. Occurs proportionately more often in stage 4 sleep

4. Not related to urinary infection
5. Individual psychotherapy indicated in most cases

DIRECTIONS: For questions 42 through 100, one or more of the alternatives given are correct. After you decide which of the alternatives are correct, record your selection according to the following key.

(A) if alternatives 1, 2, and 3 only are correct.
(B) if alternatives 1 and 3 only are correct.
(C) if alternatives 2 and 4 only are correct.
(D) if alternative 4 only is correct.
(E) if all four alternatives are correct.

42. Laboratory findings often seen in alcoholics include:

1. Increased white cell count
2. Increased mean corpuscular volume
3. Decreased blood urea
4. Increased aspartase aminotransferase

43. Correct statements about disulfiram treatment of alcoholics include:

1. Indicated where hepatic cirrhosis present
2. Used where patients do not comply with other treatment regimens
3. Preferred treatment in patients with Korsakoff's syndrome
4. May have toxic reaction with use of aftershave

44. Which of the following statements about clozapine are correct?

1. Increased salivation may be a problem
2. Frequent dystonic reactions in young males
3. Risk of agranulocytosis, especially in females
4. Retinal pigmentary changes at high therapeutic doses

45. Which of the following statements about L-tryptophan are correct?

1. Ingestion of tryptophan-rich foods increases brain serotonin
2. Metabolized by monoamine oxidase
3. Mildly sedating effect
4. Relieves early morning wakening in depressed patients

46. Which of the following would be compatible with the diagnosis of body dysmorphic disorder?

1. A 16-year-old boy who insists on a dermatological examination because of severe acne
2. A depressed middle-aged woman who believes her insides are rotting away

3. A 20-year-old man who feels he is a woman and desires anatomic sex change

4. A 25-year-old woman seeking plastic surgery for slightly prominent ears which she thinks have ruined her social life

47. Which of the following statements apply to Creutzfeldt-Jakob disease?

1. Rapidly progressive dementia
2. Onset in early adulthood
3. Fasciculations and myoclonus in limbs
4. Hereditary metabolic disorder

48. When compared with dementia subjects, patients with pseudodementia are likely to show which of the following?

1. Memory loss for specific events
2. Greater suffering and complaining about memory loss
3. Improvement after electroconvulsive therapy
4. Greater effort to perform tasks or testing

49. Potentially fatal effects of tricyclic antidepressant overdose include which of the following?

1. Ventricular arrhythmia
2. Rhabdomyolysis with renal failure
3. Respiratory depression
4. Hyperpyrexia

50. Valid statements about bulimia nervosa include which of the following?

1. Preferred weight within normal weight range
2. Scars and abrasions on back of hands
3. Ipecac abuse produces cardiomyopathy
4. High incidence of alcohol abuse

51. Which of the following statements about pregnancy and drug abuse are correct?
1. Low-dose methadone maintenance safest treatment for pregnant heroin addict
2. Opioid withdrawal liable to cause miscarriage or fetal death
3. Cocaine addiction causes increased abruptio placentae
4. Increased incidence of tricuspid valve defects in PCP abusers

52. Which of the following statements about lithium use in the elderly are correct?

1. Decreased half-life in elderly
2. Maintenance often effective at 0.4 mEq per liter
3. Safe and effective with coexisting Alzheimer's disease
4. Initial doses for mania 150–300 mg twice daily

53. Medications with pharmacologically active metabolites include:

1. Lorazepam
2. Amitriptyline
3. Lithium carbonate
4. Thioridazine

54. Which of the following would indicate childhood schizophrenia rather than autistic disorder?

1. Onset before age 5
2. Auditory and visual hallucinations
3. Mental retardation
4. Family history of schizophrenia

55. Which of the following statements about speech and language development are correct?

1. By age 18 months uses two-word phrases
2. Vocalization will differentiate hearing babies from deaf babies by age 2 months
3. Language disordered children can imitate speech sounds or noises
4. With developmental articulation disorder, retardation in vocabulary and grammar

56. Which of the following statements about postpartum women are correct?

1. Mild postpartum blues occur in 50% or more
2. Psychosis not higher after stillbirth or premature delivery
3. Bipolar patients with postpartum disorder have highest risk of recurrence
4. Patients on benzodiazepines should not breast feed

57. Which of the following disorders are associated with Down's syndrome?

1. Hypothyroidism
2. Hearing impairment
3. Alzheimer's disease
4. Male sterility

58. Which of the following statements about obsessive compulsive personality disorder are correct?

1. Character traits resemble a normal 2-year-old child
2. Increased liability to depression
3. Regressed to infantile superego
4. Episodic explosive anger

59. Which of the following statements are applicable to recently bereaved adults?

1. Depressed mood with loss of appetite and sleep disturbances
2. Increased risk of death

3. Increased morbidity with bereavement after accidental death
4. Perceived social support improves well-being

60. Since 1950, the numbers of hospitalized schizophrenics in the United States have declined due to which of
the following factors?

1. Decrease in number of schizophrenics rehospita-
lized
2. Increase in number of acute schizophrenics receiving treatment at community centers
3. Increased federal funding of hospitals for adult
mentally ill
4. Increase in chronic schizophrenics treated by community centers

61. Which of the following statements about the Fragile
X syndrome are correct?

1. Female carriers are not retarded
2. Increased incidence in autistic males
3. Testicular enlargement and long narrow face at
birth
4. High incidence of mitral valve prolapse

62. Which of the following statements about the neuroleptic malignant syndrome are correct?

1. Precipitated by levodopa withdrawal
2. Elevated creatine phosphokinase
3. Precipitated by dose increase with chronic neuroleptic use
4. Syndrome liable to recur when neuroleptic restarted

63. Which of the following statements about children
with encopresis are correct?

1. Soiling more common at night than in daytime
2. Chronic cases usually have constipation with
overflow soiling
3. No relationship with coercive training
4. Laxatives and fecal softeners useful in treatment

64. Normal behaviors in a 3-year-old child include:

1. Riding a tricycle
2. Copying a circle
3. Unbuttoning buttons
4. Taking turns

65. On a medical or surgical unit, elderly patients are
more likely to have:

1. Dystonic reactions to antipsychotic medication
2. Adverse reactions to anticholinergic drugs
3. Decreased benzodiazepine effect due to cimetidine use
4. Lithium toxicity when chlorothiazide prescribed

66. Characteristic manifestations of the neuroleptic malignant syndrome include:

1. Rhabdomyolysis
2. Temporal lobe spiking on electroencephalogram
3. Hyperpyrexia
4. Agranulocytosis

67. Which of the following statements about privilege
are correct?

1. Privilege decisions decided by physician
2. Privilege waived in mental state issue
3. Privilege is decided by patient's attorney
4. Privilege inoperable in suit against doctor

68. Increased incidence of infantile autism has been associated with:

1. Down's syndrome
2. Fragile X syndrome
3. Lesch-Nyhan syndrome
4. Infantile spasms

69. Which of the following statements about victims of
date rape are correct?

1. More likely to blame themselves
2. Less likely than other rape victims to report to police
3. Many have post-traumatic stress disorder symptoms
4. More liable to fear loss of friends' support if reports attack

70. Elderly patients are at increased risk of disabling side
effects of benzodiazepines due to:

1. Impairment of hepatic metabolism
2. Increased body fat relative to body mass
3. Reduction in renal clearance
4. Increased sensitivity to cognitive impairment

71. Which of the following are typical of seasonal affective disorder?

1. Hypersomnia, carbohydrate craving, and weight
gain
2. Predominantly in females
3. Often spring and summer hypomania
4. High family incidence of mood disorder

72. A 42-year-old psychiatric patient presents with confusion, impaired memory, and fleeting visual hallucinations. These symptoms could be side effects of:

1. Benztropine
2. Thioridazine
3. Amitriptyline
4. Atropine

73. When lithium is maintained within the usual therapeutic range, common side effects include:

    1. Seizures
    2. Dysarthria
    3. Ataxia
    4. Fine tremor

74. Which of the following statements about alcoholism
are correct?

    1. Spontaneous remission rate higher in men than in
    women
    2. Men more likely than women to develop cirrhosis
    3. Women alcoholics more likely than men alco-
    holics to have mood disorder
    4. Hospital admissions for alcoholism rise with in-
    creasing age

75. Correct statements about adolescent suicides include
which of the following?

    1. High incidence of alcohol and drug abuse
    2. Frequently precipitated by loss or humiliation
    3. Rate more than doubled in last 30 years
    4. Suicide rate rises to early adulthood and thereaf-
    ter falls gradually

76. Which of the following statements about the Tarasoff decisions are correct?

    1. Third parties warned before harm has occurred
    2. Clinicians expected to evaluate predictable dan-
    gerousness
    3. Danger causing warning must be potentially se-
    vere
    4. Confidentiality waived before dangerous behavior
    has occurred

77. Depression may be induced by:

    1. Methyldopa
    2. Reserpine
    3. Clonidine
    4. Propranolol

78. Side effects of monoamine oxidase inhibitors include:

    1. Postural hypotension
    2. Hypomania
    3. Weight gain
    4. Hyperpyrexia with meperidine

79. Medications that are effective when administered in-
tramuscularly include:

    1. Lorazepam
    2. Amitriptyline
    3. Fluphenazine
    4. Diazepam

80. When sleep terrors and nightmares are compared,
which of the following are correct?

    1. Both most common in preadolescence
    2. Both occur in stage 3-4 sleep
    3. Individual recalls nightmare, does not remember
    sleep terror
    4. Both precipitated by barbiturate withdrawal

81. Manifestations of abrupt withdrawal from chronic
opioid use include:

    1. Seizures
    2. Muscle twitching
    3. Tactile hallucinations
    4. Pupillary dilation

82. Manifestations of AIDS dementia complex are likely
to include which of the following?

    1. Elevated cerebrospinal fluid protein
    2. Generalized slowing on the electroencephalogram
    3. Cortical atrophy and reduced density of central
    white matter on MRI scan
    4. Forgetfulness, loss of concentration, and confu-
    sion

83. Which of the following are features of David Malan's
brief psychotherapy?

    1. Focus on problem at onset
    2. Duration flexible to deal with problem
    3. Interpretation of transference
    4. Avoidance of confrontation

84. Which of the following are characteristic of late onset bipolar disorder?

    1. Affects women more than men
    2. Manic symptoms likely to be severe
    3. More likely to be Type I bipolar
    4. Men more often affected than women

85. Which of the following statements about priapism
are correct?

    1. Precipitated by strong sexual arousal
    2. Requires emergency treatment
    3. Increases sexual potency
    4. Side effect of trazodone

86. Which of the following statements about the alcohol
withdrawal syndrome are correct?

    1. Even well-nourished patients should be given thi-
    amine
    2. Patients likely to be overhydrated rather than de-
    hydrated
    3. Long-acting benzodiazepines in tapered doses
    during acute stages
    4. Intramuscular chlorpromazine for disruptive
    symptoms

Case number 87–88

87–88. A 21-year-old woman is brought for examination. Her mother says the patient hardly eats at all and has lost 30 pounds in the last six months. The patient is very verbal, admits that she has lost weight, but says that she has no problem. She is not depressed, and shows no evidence of thinking problems.

87. You will want to ask especially about:

1. Cessation of menses
2. Laxative use
3. Exercising and jogging
4. Self-induced vomiting

88. Physical findings you might anticipate include:

1. Loss of body pigmentation
2. Patchy loss of scalp hair
3. Temperature elevation
4. Fine hair on arms and legs

89. Correct statements about narcolepsy include:

1. Catalepsy triggered by intense emotions
2. Symptomatic improvement with methylphenidate
3. Symptoms tend to lessen or disappear with age
4. Marked familial tendency

90. Characteristics of bipolar patients who are rapid cyclers include:

1. Four or more episodes of mania or depression each year
2. Rapid cycling typically starts with onset of illness
3. More commonly female patients
4. Likely to respond well to lithium

91. Side effects of lithium therapy include:

1. Exacerbation of psoriasis
2. Development of acne
3. Hair loss
4. Patchy skin depigmentation

92. Which of the following procedures would be appropriate in managing a patient who produces a gun in the course of emergency evaluation?

1. Ask about his or her concerns
2. Offer food
3. Move slowly and deliberately
4. Always be sure to look the patient directly in the eye

93. During cocaine withdrawal, which of the following symptoms should be anticipated?

1. Grand mal convulsions in the first three days
2. Hallucinations of insects crawling under the skin
3. Coronary artery spasms
4. Restlessness and agitation

94. Valid statements about children with functional enuresis include:

1. Subjects wet during all stages of sleep
2. Most have first-degree relative with history of enuresis
3. Conditioning devices often are successful
4. Psychotherapy recommended for most subjects

95. Which of the following statements about electroconvulsive therapy are correct?

1. Mood-congruent depressive delusions tend to respond well
2. Poorer response with double depression than with uncomplicated depression
3. Effect on catatonic schizophrenics equal to neuroleptic efficacy
4. Mortality rate similar to rate for brief general anesthesia

96. Which of the following statements about paranoid personality disorder are correct?

1. Unlikely to seek treatment voluntarily
2. Fixed systematic delusions
3. Undue sensitivity to fantasied slights
4. High risk of impulsive self-destructive behavior

97. Disorders more common in females include:

1. Functional encopresis
2. Elective mutism
3. Infantile autism
4. Somatization disorder

98. According to Eugene Bleuler, the fundamental symptoms of schizophrenia are:

1. Ambivalence
2. Associations loosened
3. Affect inappropriate
4. Aggression poorly controlled

99. Which of the following are likely to apply to a patient with phenylketonuria?

1. Musty odor to urine
2. Dermatitis
3. Retardation in siblings
4. Hydrocephalus

100. Which of the following statements about the Thematic Apperception Test are correct?

1. Blank card included in test series
2. Colored cards at end of set
3. Prompts information about family relationships
4. Easily scored by nonprofessional

ANSWERS AND EXPLANATIONS

1. (4) Disulfiram, an important adjunct in the treatment of alcoholism, inhibits liver microsome enzymes, and therefore may raise blood levels of phenytoin and isoniazid, resulting in intoxication. It may be necessary to adjust the dosage of oral anticoagulants since disulfiram may prolong prothrombin time. (*CTP 631, 698, 1665. APA 326. Har 707.*)

2. (4) Holmes and Rahe found a relationship between psychiatric symptoms and life stresses. They assigned point values (100 to 11) to various life changes (43). Eighty percent of those with 300 points accumulated in a year were at risk of a medical problem (e.g., accident, illness, destructive behavior), whereas subjects with an accumulated score of 200 were likely to have a psychosomatic disorder within the next several months. (*APA 496. CTP 300. Har 398–99.*)

SOME ELEMENTS OF THE SOCIAL READJUSTMENT RATING SCALE

Life Events (43 in number)	Mean Value (Points)
# 1 Death of a spouse	100
# 2 Divorce	73
#12 Pregnancy	40
#32 Change in residency	20
#41 Vacation	15
#43 Minor violations of the law, (i.e., traffic ticket)	11

3. (3) Serial 7's is a formal test for concentration. Serial 3's or counting backwards from 20 can be substituted if the patient has cognitive difficulties in performing serial 7's. Concentration reflects the patient's ability to focus and maintain his or her attention to a task. (*CTP 145. APA 191.*)

4. (1) Heinz Kohut (1971) argued that the diagnosis of narcissistic personality disorder could only be made on the basis of the emerging transferential relationship in psychoanalytic psychotherapy. He also attributed the disorder to a developmental arrest resulting from childhood disappointments and a parental failure in empathy. Kernberg stated that narcissistic grandiosity is a defensive and pathological reaction to feelings of rage and inferiority and must be confronted and interpreted rather than supported. (*CTP 366–67. APA 633. Har 191–92.*)

5. (5) *Akathisia* ("restless legs") is an extrapyramidal disorder manifested by an unpleasant feeling of motor restlessness, with fidgeting, pacing, and an inability to sit still. Akathisia is among the most treatment-refractory extrapyramidal symptoms. The treatment of choice is the beta-adrenergic blocking drugs, particu-larly propranolol. Benzodiazepines or amantadine may be effective. (*APA 779–80. CTP 1624. Har 495.*)

6. (2) *Alexithymia*. The inability to recognize or describe one's emotional feelings in words, often with a limited fantasy life and a general constriction in the affective life. It can be seen in patients with post-traumatic stress disorder, addiction, or psychosomatic problems.

   Anhedonia. The inability to experience pleasure from activities that produce normally pleasurable feelings.

   Aphasia. A deficit of language, which may be due to motor or sensory dysfunction, resulting in the loss of the ability to speak or comprehend the meaning of written or printed words and sentences (neurological problem).

   Alexia. A loss of power to grasp the meaning of written or printed words and sentences (neurological problem).

   Dyslexia. An inability or difficulty in reading, often with a tendency to reverse letters and words in reading and writing. (*CTP 573. APA 1240. Har 104–8, 390.*)

7. (4) Stimulants have the following common side effects—anorexia, weight loss, abdominal pain, irritability and insomnia. Tics, Tourette's disorder, hypertension, psychosis, and cardiovascular problems may be induced or worsened. With stimulant overdose, death can occur from fever, cardiovascular shock, and convulsions. Stimulant medications can decrease hyperactivity, or disruptive behavior, and improve cognitive tasks (attention, distractibility, impulsivity, short-term memory). There is no apparent effect on learning disabilities without ADHD. Mild dysphoria can occur after stopping stimulants. (*APA 990–93. CTP 1835–36. Har 419.*)

8. (4) Thiamine (vitamin B_1) deficiency, most commonly caused by alcoholism, is believed to be the cause of Wernicke-Korsakoff's syndrome, which is manifested by delirium, encephalopathy, truncal ataxia, ophthalmoplegia (especially sixth cranial nerve), nystagmus, mental confusion, amnestic disorder, and in some cases, death. (*CTP 620. APA 323. Har 363, 709.*)

9. (4) The first sign of impending puberty in girls related to increased estrogen levels is breast development (breast buds) with increase in size and pigmentation of areolae and nipple. (*CTP 1332–33. Har 640–41. APA 113–14.*)

10. (4) Homosexual rape is more frequent among men than women and occurs primarily in closed institutions, such

as hospitals and prisons. The male victims feel the same as females who have been raped (shame, guilt, depression)—they feel that they have been ruined, they blame themselves, and they fear they will become homosexual. Many develop sexual dysfunction problems. (*CTP 1099.*)

11. **(5)** Heinz Kohut (1913–1981) developed the psychoanalytic school of "self-psychology." He described three new concepts of transference related to narcissistic and self-object relations: mirroring, idealizing, and alter ego. He stressed that the paramount need for psychoanalysis is to operate on the basis of empathy. (*CTP 1452. Har 192. APA 142.*)

12. **(2)** During the postpartum period, 20–40% of mothers report emotional disturbance or cognitive dysfunctions ("postpartum blues"), consisting of sadness, dysphoria, frequent tearfulness, and clinging dependency. This is different from the more rare postpartum psychosis (1–2 per 1,000 deliveries), which is characterized by severe anxiety, depression, and hallucinations with or without delusions. Postpartum blues can occur in fathers, but less frequently. There is an increased risk for postpartum psychosis if the mother had previous postpartum psychosis, mood disorder, or organic brain syndrome (from infections, toxemia). The psychosis occurs within 30 days of birth in primiparas but earlier postpartum occurs with subsequent deliveries. Patients with postpartum psychosis have a higher risk of suicide (5%) and of infanticide (4%). (*CTP 852–58, 1219.*)

13. **(3)** "*Respondeat superior*" is the legal principle that requires the supervisor of a trainee to be responsible for the care of the patient, and to inform the patient of the training and supervisory status of the relationship.

"*Parens patriae*," "father of his country," is the power of the state to commit or protect individuals who may cause harm to themselves or others.

"*Mens rea*" means evil intent and is one component of an objectionable act under criminal law. The other is "actus reus," voluntary conduct.

"*Res ipsa loquitur*" refers to the fact that the thing or act speaks for itself. (*CTP 2111. Har 800.*)

14. **(2)** To render a professional opinion based on a political matter and not on a clinical evaluation could be considered unethical. "Primum non nocere," first do no harm, is the backbone of the Hippocratic tradition. The AMA developed a code of ethics in 1847 with many revisions since, and the APA incorporated these in 1981 and 1985. These codes delineate physicians' responsibilities to society—to be respectful of the rights of others, to be competent in professional skills, and to be honest in dealing with others. (*APA 1085–86. Har 798.*)

15. **(4)** *Prevalence rate* is the frequency or proportion of a disorder at a given point (point prevalence) or period of time.

Concordance rate, used in genetic studies, refers to the similarity in a pair of related individuals with respect to presence or absence of a disease or trait.

Specificity rate is the number of true cases or noncases who are accurately assessed by an instrument.

Incidence rate is the number of new cases during a specific period of time.

Relative risk is the ratio of the incidence rates of two groups, usually those with a disorder and those exposed but without the disorder. (*CTP 314–15. APA 1274–75. Har 762.*)

16. **(2)** Benzodiazepines have antianxiety, sedative, anticonvulsive, and muscle relaxant properties, and are effective as a preoperative sedative. Only three benzodiazepines have parental preparations—chlordiazepoxide, diazepam, and lorazepam. Intramuscular administration is not advisable except for lorazepam. (*APA 812. CTP 1580–83. Har 526–27.*)

17. **(3)** Tourette's disorder has three main characteristics: (1) motor tics in neck, face, and sometimes lower limbs; (2) vocal tics, which can range from throat clearing to snorting, barking, swearing, and profanity (coprolalia); and (3) obsessive compulsive symptomatology. Onset of Tourette's disorder is usually age 2 to 13 years. (*CTP 1865–78. APA 686. Har 123.*)

18. **(4)** *Reactive attachment disorder* of infancy and early childhood (before age 5) covers a broad range of conditions and etiologies. Basically, it is a failure to thrive emotionally and physically, secondary to grossly inadequate caregiving. Lengthy institutionalizations and hospitalizations or frequent changes in primary caretaker as in multiple foster home placements may be a cause for the disorder. The essential feature is markedly disturbed social relatedness. (*CTP 1894–1903. Har 626.*)

19. **(2)** Children with Down's syndrome tend to have an IQ under 50, although there are many exceptions. Most are educable (IQs 40 and above) and trainable (IQs between 20–40). The general belief that these children are lovable, docile, and cheerful is not always accurate, but this perception helps in their placement in foster care and adoptive families. (*CTP 1739–41. Har 685.*)

20. **(2)** Compulsive gamblers are risk takers who fail to profit from their gambling misadventures. They are described as competitive, independent, overconfident, and unduly optimistic. Gamblers Anonymous is patterned after Alcoholics Anonymous. Pathological gambling and alcoholism are more common in fathers of

males and mothers of females with the disorder, and these subjects are thus exposed to gambling early in life. Major affective disorders (32%) and alcoholism (36%) occur in first-degree relatives. When compulsive gamblers abruptly stop gambling (i.e., when hospitalized), they develop withdrawal symptoms similar to substance abusers. (*CTP 1146–47. APA 613–15.*)

21. (4) *Primary prevention* is the avoidance or elimination of the occurrence of an illness, as with eradication of the causative factors.

Secondary prevention involves case finding and treatment to minimize and prevent permanent disability and to regain normal functioning after an illness has developed.

Tertiary prevention is rehabilitation of the residual defect in order to reduce and limit the degree or sequelae of the disability. (*CTP 2067–71. APA 1155. Har 783.*)

22. (2) Increased risk of toxic effects is associated with daily doses of 300 mg or over of imipramine and effects include cardiovascular toxicity, psychotic agitation, and confusion. Postural hypotension is probably the most common cardiovascular side effect. With overdose, there is a potential risk of malignant ventricular arrhythmias, cardiac arrest, syncope, or congestive heart failure. Although ECG changes on lower doses are common and include tachycardia, prolongation of the Q-T intervals, and flattening of the T-waves, the quinidine-like effect of imipramine at therapeutic plasma levels may actually reduce the number of premature ventricular contractions. (*CTP 1644–48. APA 799–800. Har 512.*)

23. (3) *Privilege* is provided to the patient not to the psychiatrist. A physician may not reveal the confidences entrusted to him or her in the course of medical attendance, except when required by law, to protect the welfare of an individual or community, or when the patient revokes or releases the privilege. (*CTP 2119–20. Har 824–25.*)

24. (5) Transference reactions occur in all relationships, including doctor-patient encounters. Transference can be positive, which usually facilitates a patient's efforts to communicate but it can be too intense, can be a barrier, and may result in resistant and negative behavior. The working collaboration between therapist and patient is based on a therapeutic alliance and involves the patient's conscious and unconscious desires to cooperate. (*CTP 1446–48. Har 14–16.*)

25. (2) In the general population, suicide is the ninth to tenth leading cause of death nationally (10–12/ 100,000), second or third for white males ages 15–19 years, and first for physicians under 40 years. Half of

the male suicides are by firearms, but this is a factor in only one-quarter of female suicides. Although the rate of adolescent and young adult suicide has more than doubled since 1960, the highest rate of suicide is in elderly males (over 65). Increased risk factors for suicide are single, divorced, living alone, depression (especially with previous suicide attempts), schizophrenia, and substance abuse (especially alcoholism). (*CTP 1414–26. Har 743. APA 1023–25.*)

26. (2) Impotence can be caused by medical (organic) or psychogenic factors. Major organic causes of sexual dysfunction for both males and females are: diabetic, liver, renal, and cardiovascular diseases; pain and surgery; endocrine disorders, especially hypothyroidism and hypopituitarism; infectious mononucleosis; substances, such as alcohol, sedatives, stimulants (especially cocaine, amphetamines), narcotics, neuroleptics (especially thioridazine, fluphenazine), and antihypertensive drugs. Trazodone may infrequently cause priapism, a medical emergency if an erection lasts more than one hour: untreated priapism can result in impotence. (*CTP 1051–53, 1647. Har 569–71.*)

27. (1) Psychiatric experts can act as a nontestifying consultants, or can be called upon to testify at deposition and trial. They may be asked by the court to testify on the issue of competency, testamentary capacity, diagnosis, treatment, or criminal responsibility. Expert witnesses are permitted to offer opinions not allowed by other witnesses and may be asked to comment on hearsay evidence. (*CTP 2122–23. APA 1077, 1272.*)

28. (3) *Placebo effect* occurs when a response to medications is due to a psychological effect and not to a pharmacological action. Placebos do have definite therapeutic and side effects in a significant percentage of patients. There are many poorly understood factors of patients' responses to physicians and placebos, which are referred to as nonspecific therapeutic factors. Problems of anxiety, pain, and general recovery can be seen with the use of a placebo. The use of a placebo may cause a problem with trust: the patient may feel manipulated or betrayed. (*CTP 1289, 1686.*)

29. (4) *Sleep apnea* is a common condition, particularly with obese males over age 40, and is usually caused by repeated cessation of breathing during the night due to obstruction to the airflow (also causing loud snoring). A CNS disorder rarely causes sleep apnea. Daytime sleepiness and hypertension are commonly associated conditions. Treatment may include weight loss, sleeping on one side, use of tongue retaining devices, continuous positive airway pressure or even a modified tracheotomy (uvulopalatopharyngoplasty). (*CTP 1115. Har 166. APA 745–46.*)

30. (4) *Blocking* is a sudden obstruction or interruption in spontaneous flow of thinking or speaking.

> *Thought insertion* is the subjective experience that thoughts are being inserted into one's consciousness by some outside agency.
>
> *Dissociation* is the splitting off of mental contents from conscious awareness, the separation of an idea from its emotional affect.
>
> *Suppression* is the conscious effort to control and conceal unacceptable thoughts, feelings, or impulses.
>
> *Isolation* is a mechanism of defense in which the affect of an idea is kept unconscious leaving the conscious idea neutral. (*CTP 375. APA 1248. Har 268.*)

31. (5) *Elective mutism* is an unusual childhood disorder in that the disorder is more common in girls than in boys. (*CTP 1887–89.*)

32. (4) *Object permanence* is the critical achievement during the sensorimotor main stage (birth to 2 years) where the child is able to differentiate between himself or herself and the world, is able to maintain a mental image, and can understand that objects have their own existence even though they are not present or visible.

> *Conservation*, as a thinking ability, develops during the concrete operational stage (ages 7–14 years).
>
> *Object constancy* is present when a toddler has a permanent, stable image of the whole object. (*CTP 258. Har 609. APA 100–101.*)

33. (3) During the first ten years of a bipolar disorder, episodes become more frequent, but later in life, episodes tend to become fewer. (*CTP 893–94. APA 413.*)

34. (3) Bulimia patients have problems with depression, high anxiety, compulsivity, chemical dependency (especially alcohol), impulsive stealing or shoplifting, and suicidal behaviors. (*CTP 1860. APA 760. Har 436.*)

35. (2) Primary care physicians (defined as general practitioners, family medicine, internists, and pediatricians) make up about 35% of all doctors. Psychiatrists constitute about 6% of the total, and tend to be concentrated in major urban cities. Some studies indicate that up to 28% of patient visits to a general physician were because of a diagnosable mental disorder. NIMH studies estimate that 60% of mental health care is in the general health care sector, whereas only 20% is by a private or public mental health care professional. (*CTP 1280–81. APA 80. Har 788.*)

36. (4) *Generativity*, the ability to create, is part of productive adulthood (40–65 years).

> *Integrity*—wisdom, comfort and continued involvement—evolves in later adulthood (over 65 years).
>
> *Intimacy versus isolation* is the task of early, mature adulthood (20–40 years).
>
> *Industry*, channeled learning, develops from age 7 to early adolescence. (*CTP 405–8. Har 613.*)

37. (5) The *Ganser syndrome*, sometimes called a pseudodementia, is rare and is referred to as a "syndrome of approximate answers." It is usually seen in persons facing a stressful life situation, but who are attempting to escape responsibilities or to evade the problem. (*CTP 1139. APA 582. Har 377.*)

38. (1) *Kappa statistic* or technique is used for quantifying diagnostic reliability and categorical judgments, indexing agreement among clinicians, and correcting for chance agreement. The values range from -1.0 (total disagreement) to +1.0 (perfect agreement), with 0 indicating no more than chance agreement. A value of .70 and above is good, .50 to .70 is fair, and below .50 is poor. (*CTP 312–14. Har 74. APA 207.*)

39. (3) *Acute opioid overdose* can be immediately treated by the opioid antagonists naltrexone (long-acting) and naloxone (short-acting). These drugs can also precipitate withdrawal symptoms. Other medications of value in detoxification from narcotics are clonidine and methadone. Abusers may be dependent on several substances, which can have different withdrawal symptoms, all of which require treatment. (*CTP 656–57. APA 336. Har 711.*)

40. (3) *Regression* is a return to a more infantile or earlier level of maturational functioning.

> *Repression* is the unconscious defense whereby unwanted affects, memories, or drives are kept from consciousness.
>
> *Castration anxiety* is due to a fantasied danger or injury to body or genitals.
>
> *Reaction formation* is the defense mechanism where affects are expressed in the manner opposite to the underlying unacceptable emotions.
>
> *Autism* is a pervasive developmental disorder with many severe disturbances in physical, social, adaptive, and language areas. (*APA 136, 1245. Har 217, 222. CTP 375–6.*)

41. (2) Functional enuresis is common, more frequent in males, runs in families, and 80% is primary (individuals have never attained bladder control). (*CTP 1879–82. APA 690–91.*)

42. (C) Laboratory findings in alcoholism may show the following: blood gamma-glutamyltransferase (GTT) increased in greater than 50% of alcoholics, and in 80%

with liver problems; increased uric acid, triglycerides, aspartase aminotransferase, and urea; increased mean corpuscular volume, decreased white blood cell count; and EEGs nonspecific slowing in intoxication, but also seen in overdose of sedative hypnotics.

Biological markers for alcoholism are nonspecific as yet. (*APA 320.*)

43. **(D)** Disulfiram (Antabuse) competitively inhibits the enzyme aldehyde dehydrogenase so that alcohol intake in a person taking disulfiram causes a toxic reaction due to acetaldehyde accumulation in the blood. The reactions are flushing and feelings of heat in the face, sclera, upper limbs, and chest; becoming pale, hypotensive, nauseated, and experiencing severe malaise, dizziness, blurred vision, palpitations, air hunger, and numbness of extremities. The most serious alcohol disulfiram reactions are severe hypotension, respiratory depression, cardiovascular collapse, unconsciousness, convulsions, and death.

Treatment is to use general supportive means, vitamin C in massive doses IV (one gram), and ephedrine sulfate. Potassium blood levels must be monitored. Antihistamines may be helpful. (*CTP 687, 698. APA 326. Har 706–8.*)

44. **(B)** Clozapine (Clozaril) is a dibenzodiazepine antipsychotic medication and is different from clonazepam (Klonopin, an anticonvulsant benzodiazepine). Clozapine is associated with agranulocytosis. It lacks parkinsonian side effects associated with most antipsychotics. (*CTP 1618. Har 147, 488.*)

45. **(B)** The amino acid precursor tryptophan is converted into serotonin (5-hydroxytryptamine). One to six grams is an effective hypnotic dose, which can be obtained from a large glass of milk. One to fifteen grams of tryptophan reduce sleep latency and nocturnal awakening. L-tryptophan deficiency is associated with less time in REM sleep. In newborns, adding L-tryptophan to formula hastens the onset of both REM and NREM sleep. Valine competes with L-tryptophan for entry into brain and prolongs onset of both sleep states. Tryptophan has been taken off the market following reports of fatal reactions: it is not known whether tryptophan itself or some contaminant is the cause of these reactions. (*CTP 49, 1591. APA 818. Har 160.*)

46. **(D)** *Body dysmorphic disorder*, also known as dysmorphophobia, is present when patients think they are physically defective in some way even though they have no outward appearance problem. This body dislike is not on the level of a delusion, as these patients can acknowledge that their feelings may be exaggerated. The disorder can coexist with schizophrenia, mood disorders, or severe personality disorders. (*CTP 1025–27.*)

47. **(B)** *Creutzfeldt-Jakob disease*, a very rare disorder with one new case per million general population per year, is caused by a slow virus, which has no immune response, and is difficult to inactivate. The disease appears during ages 40–60, starting with mild dementia, myoclonic jerks, and fasciculations. After the diagnosis is made, a rapid downhill course typically ensues with severe dementia and death in months to a year. Pathological changes show widespread spongiform changes, neuronal loss, and cytoplasmic vacuolation in the central nervous system. (*CTP 187–88. APA 289–90.*)

48. **(A)** Comparison of pseudodementia (also called "the dementia syndrome of depression") and dementia (*CTP 621–23. APA 297–98. Har 672–73.*)

	Pseudodementia	Dementia
Onset:	weeks	months
Duration of SxS:	months	years
Loss of social skills:	early	late
Effort to cope:	poor	good
Mood:	depressed	unconcerned
Cognition:	preserved	faulty
Motivation:	poor	tries
Orientation:	fair	mistakes
Memory:	gaps	no gaps
Response to testing:	highlights failure	pleased with success
Physical:	normal	problems
Antidepression treatment:	improves	may worsen

49. **(B)** Because tricyclic antidepressants (HCA) are metabolized in the liver, drugs that induce hepatic microsomal enzymes will result in decreased plasma levels (i.e., alcohol, anticonvulsants, barbiturates, chloral hydrate, glutethimide, oral contraceptives, and cigarettes).

Increased plasma levels of HCAs can be induced by antipsychotic drugs, methylphenidate, and increasing age.

The major complications from overdose of HCAs are neuropsychiatric impairment (agitation, delirium), hypotension, cardiac arrhythmias, and seizures. These toxic effects can lead to coma and death. (*CTP 1647–48. APA 801–2. Har 514–17.*)

50. **(E)** *Bulimia* ("ox hunger") refers to binge eating. The individual's weight in controlled by self-induced vomiting, dieting and less frequently by laxative use. A minority of bulimics use diuretics. Only one-third to one-fifth of bulimic individuals are mildly overweight before start of episodes, and most choose to maintain a normal weight range throughout the disorder. The majority of patients have depressive symptoms, interpersonal relations problems, impulsivity, high levels of anxiety, and compulsions. Substance abuse is not uncommon, especially with alcohol. Impulsive stealing

(food, clothing, jewelry) may be present before the on-set of binge eating.

Electrolyte abnormalities lead to weakness, lethargy, and at times cardiac arrhythmias and even cardiac arrest.

Erosion and severe attrition of teeth, parotid gland enlargement, acute dilation of stomach, and esophageal tears can occur due to vomiting. "Russell's sign" is manifested by the abrasions and scars on the backs of hands from persistent efforts to self-induce vomiting. Emetine (ipecac) intoxication can cause a cardiomyopathy with resultant cardiac failure. During emetine abuse, there are changing laboratory findings usually showing increasing liver enzymes and erythrocyte sedimentation rate, which should alert the physician to this problem. (*CTP 1854–64. APA 760–63.*)

51. (A) Pregnant women using cocaine have increased rates of abruptio placenta. Their babies have decreased interactive behavior as measured on the Brazelton scale. HIV positive mothers, usually infected from IV opioid addiction, are likely to have HIV positive babies. Sixty-eight to ninety-four percent of neonates born to heroin addicts develop a syndrome of narcotic withdrawal: these infants show a total perinatal mortality as high as 10.7%, with 4% stillbirths and 6.7% neonatal deaths. Withdrawal problems are improved if mother is in a supervised methadone maintenance program.

Maternal alcohol abuse can result in a fetal alcohol syndrome, which consists of decreased birth weight, growth retardation before or after birth, abnormal features of face and head (small head circumference, flattening of facial features), and mental retardation. Smoking (nicotine) during pregnancy results in decreased birth weight. (*CTP 684–85. APA 319, 331, 340, 350.*)

52. (C) Lithium treatment in the elderly should start with low doses (300–600 mg/day in divided doses). Doses larger than 900 mg/day generally are not needed. Renal filtration (main route of excretion) decreases with increasing age, thereby increasing blood levels. Prolonged lithium treatment in the elderly can cause subtle forms of an organic mental disorder (i.e., delirium or reversible dementia). (*CTP 2044–45. APA 1132–33. Har 505.*)

53. (C) Commonly used medications with pharmacologically active metabolites are amitriptyline, thioridazine, diazepam, and chlordiazepoxide. (*CTP 1580, 1593, 1643–44.*)

54. (C) *Autism* is usually apparent in infancy or early childhood. Autism is a subdivision of pervasive developmental disorder with no specific thought disorder (i.e., hallucinations or delusions).

Whereas schizophrenics have autistic (i.e., idiosyncratic) thinking, their premorbid functioning is on higher levels than autistic patients; onset is most often in late adolescence or young adulthood manifested by a thought disorder (hallucinations, delusions). Schizophrenics have a higher family incidence of schizophrenia. Higher family incidence of schizophrenia is not typical of autistic patients. (*CTP 1979. APA 367, 714–15. Har 281–82, 716.*)

55. (B) Speech and language development are related to cognitive development and are important milestones. Delayed speech in a child should motivate parents to seek professional help. The child progresses from noises (four weeks) to "mama, dada" (40 weeks), to six words at 52 weeks, 10–19 words at 15 months, 20–29 words at 18 months, and over 50 words plus three to four word sentences at 24 months. Children can imitate smiles and simple sounds at 16 weeks and more complex sounds after 40 weeks. (*CTP 1812–17. APA 99. Har 688.*)

56. (E) In the postpartum period, about 20–40% of mothers report emotional disturbances or cognitive dysfunction, and many experience "postpartum blues," feeling sad and tearful. Postpartum blues can also occur with fathers. Postpartum psychosis is rare and occurs in 1–2 per 1,000 deliveries. Many medications can be passed in the breast milk to the nursing infant. (*CTP 852–58, 1219.*)

57. (E) *Down's syndrome*, trisomy 21, has the chromosome 21 gene for beta-amyloid, which is accumulated in the neuritic plaques. If the individual lives to age 35, he or she is likely to show neurofibrillary tangibles and progressive neuropathological changes similar to Alzheimer's disease. Other problems seen in Down's syndrome patients besides mental retardation include hypotonia, cardiac anomalies, hearing problems, seizures, hypothyroidism, and sterility. (*CTP 614, 1739–41. APA 708. Har 370.*)

58. (A) The essential features of *obsessive compulsive personality disorder* are inflexibility, rigidity, perfectionism, and excessive preoccupation with control and orderliness. These subjects have problems with expressing warmth and tender emotions. Major defense mechanisms utilized are based on the preoedipal infantile superego, anal-sadistic phase, including reaction formation, rationalization, and undoing. Individuals with this disorder are prone to depression especially in middle age or older. (*CTP 984–99. Har 352–53. APA 640–41.*)

59. (E) Uncomplicated bereavement, grief (conscious impact of loss), and mourning (reactive process of coping with loss) begin immediately or within a few weeks af-

ter a death or loss and are manifested by many symptoms, including sadness, preoccupation about the deceased, guilt, insomnia, difficulty in concentration, anger, hostility, tearfulness, and somatic distress. Usually the normal mourning process is completed in six months (often determined by culture). Guilt is likely to be a more serious problem when there is a sudden death, such as stillbirth, sudden infant death, cardiac arrest, death after surgery, murder, suicide, accidental or traumatic death especially if disfigurement is present. Most societies have rituals such as wakes, funerals and burial services that help the process of mourning. (*CTP 1339. APA 1130. Har 747–50.*)

60. **(C)** The rate of new cases (incidence) of schizophrenia admitted to hospitals is increasing. The duration of hospitalization has decreased despite the increased number of new admissions as more inpatients are transferred to outpatient clinics. The number of children born to schizophrenics has doubled over the past twenty years. Schizophrenics (especially those age 65 and older) still utilize a disproportionate share of general medical and psychiatric services. (*CTP 2083–90. Har 281. APA 378.*)

61. **(C)** *Fragile X chromosome syndrome* is a common disorder in males (1/1,000) and the second most common genetic cause of moderate and severe mental retardation (Down's is the first). Affected males have large testes after puberty (macro-orchidism), large jaw, forehead, ears and head circumference, mitral valve prolapse (80%), hyperextensible joints, high arched palate, and autistic features (20–40%). About 10% of autistic males have Fragile X syndrome. (*CTP 1741–42. APA 708.*)

62. **(E)** *Neuroleptic malignant syndrome* can occur any time during treatment with antipsychotic agents, and the mechanism is unknown. The symptoms consist of hyperthermia, severe extrapyramidal effects, "lead pipe" muscle rigidity, autonomic dysfunction, clouded consciousness (i.e., delirium, coma), leukocytosis (greater than 15,000 WBCs), and increased creatinine phosphokinase (greater than 300 U/ml). The mortality rate can be from 15 to 25%. (*CTP 1624–25. APA 783–84. Har 495–96.*)

63. **(C)** *Functional encopresis* during the daytime is much more frequent than nocturnal encopresis. In one-half of cases, bowel control has not yet been achieved (i.e., primary). Secondary encopresis (continent for at least one year, then restarts soiling) usually begins by 8 years of age. Common problems seen in encopresis are chronic constipation (with overflow incontinence), large stools, fecal impaction, stomachaches, and in girls, urinary tract problems. Physical treatment is by decompaction, utilizing bowel cleaning agents (ene-

mas), laxatives (mineral oil), and stool softeners. There is a higher incidence of encopresis in families of encopretics (but it is not considered genetic), mental retardation, medical conditions (thyroid disorders), neurodevelopmental delays, and a variety of stress-related factors (most often issues of autonomy and control). (*APA 668–70. CTP 1883–86.*)

64. **(E)** Development in children can be remembered by the mnemonic "Think SMALL": "S" stands for social-personal, "M" for motor-neurological, "A" for adaptive-coping, "L" for language and speech, and "L" for learning-intelligence.

A normal 3-year-old can do many complex tasks:

"Social"—fully toilet trained, takes turns, plays with other children, puts on shoes, unbuttons buttons, feeds self, washes and dries hands, knows front and back

"Motor"—alternates feet on stairs, throws ball overhand, builds a ten-block tower, rides a tricycle (actually starts at 30 months)

"Adaptive"—copies vertical, horizontal, circle, and cross

"Language"—uses "and" and "but," recites all of a song, knows up and down, follows three commands, knows two colors

(*APA 99–100. CTP 1702.*)

65. **(C)** *Delirium* is common, especially in the elderly, with many causes, including metabolic disorders, infections, postoperative states, intoxications (alcohol, sedatives, anticholinergics, opiates, stimulants, digitalis), drug withdrawal states, and neurological disorders (e.g., seizures, head trauma, hypertension, encephalopathy, focal disease). Drug toxicity causing delirium can result from routine doses of prescribed drugs. (*CTP 1581, 1668–69. Har 363.*)

66. **(B)** Muscle breakdown (rhabdomyolysis) causes elevated CPK, which can lead to myoglobulinuria and to acute renal failure. (See question number 62 reference NMS.) (*CTP 1624–25. APA 783–84. Har 495–96.*)

67. **(C)** *Privilege* is provided to the patient by law, not to the physician. Under privilege, the patient can prohibit the physician from revealing confidential information. If the patient waives privilege, the physician has no legal privilege for refusing to testify. (Refer to question 23.) (*CTP 2119–20. Har 824–25.*)

68. **(C)** A higher incidence of autism is associated with Fragile X syndrome and infantile spasms. When patients present with autistic symptoms, the following conditions should be considered: phenylketonuria, deafness, and mental retardation. (*CTP 1772–84. APA 715–16.*)

69. **(E)** Rape is commonly not reported by the victim despite the fact that about half of the rapists are known and 7% are close relatives. Victims are afraid to report as they often blame themselves and fear rejection by family and friends. Victims can be any age, with the greatest danger to females ages 10–29 years. Women may experience reactions of shame, fear, confusion, humiliation, and rage, all of which can last a year or longer. Post-traumatic stress disorder is not uncommon. (*CTP 1098–99.*)

70. **(E)** Elderly patients are more sensitive to the side effects of benzodiazepines. They become more sedated and dependent at lower doses, and more likely to appear demented due to medication-induced confusion, decline in memory, agitation, and disinhibition. Shorter-acting benzodiazepines are better tolerated. The elderly are prone to drug accumulation with longer-acting benzodiazepines because of delayed clearance due to age-related increased adipose tissue, less efficient metabolism, higher incidence of liver disease, and other metabolic problems. (*CTP 2039–41. Har 677–78. APA 1135.*)

71. **(E)** *Seasonal affective disorder* (SAD), also called seasonal mood disorder, occurs most often in females age 20–30. Depressions usually start in October and November, end in early spring, and manifest by hypersomnia (oversleeping), anergia (fatigue), overeating (especially craving carbohydrates), and weight gain. During early spring and summer these subjects may develop hypomania. (*CTP 923–24, 1685–86. APA 415. Har 766.*)

72. **(E)** Most neuroleptics, antidepressants, and anticholinergics have sedative side effects that are dose-related. These side effects can create problems if the patient is susceptible, has an underlying medical disease, or is taking other medications that can interact. (*CTP 1666.*)

73. **(D)** The common side effects of lithium at therapeutic blood levels are fine resting hand tremors (about 50%), anorexia, nausea, polyuria, weight gain, and leukocytosis. Problems that can occur at levels about 1.5 mEq/l include severe vomiting, ataxia, nystagmus, muscle weakness, convulsions, delirium, stupor, coma, and even death (greater than 2.5 mEq/l). (*CTP 1660. APA 821–26. Har 504–5.*)

74. **(B)** Alcoholism is the third largest health problem in the U.S., after heart disease and cancer. Medical problems related to alcohol abuse include gastrointestinal difficulties, liver dysfunction (fatty liver, cirrhosis), increased infections, blackouts, seizures, increased suicidal potential, depression, anxiety, sexual and sleep problems, and increased incidence of accidents and injuries. Males are more likely to have alcoholism than females, even though women have two times the rate of depression. Onset of problems with alcohol is later in life for females compared with males, but spontaneous remissions are less likely with females than with males. Males tend to remit in their 50s and 60s when alcoholism is most common with females. Lifetime alcoholism expectancy rate is 3–5% for males and 1% for females. (*CTP 692. APA 318. Har 701.*)

75. **(A)** Suicide is the third leading cause of death in adolescents ages 15–24 years and seventh in 5–14-year age group. Between 1960–1980, suicide rates of adolescents, mainly white males, increased 150% and in some cities even more, whereas rates for older ages (except elderly) decreased or remained stable (rates decrease during adulthood and rise again in the elderly). Adolescents who commit suicide are more likely to have been depressed, had problems with alcohol or substance abuse, and shown long-standing behavior difficulties. (*CTP 1991–92. Har 651–52. APA 1029–30.*)

76. **(E)** In the Tarasoff case, in 1974, the California Supreme Court ruled that the therapist had a legal duty to warn others or protect the intended victim. This was later modified by legislation to where a reasonable effort to communicate the threat to victim or law enforcement was acceptable. This court action, and legislation concerning the therapist's responsibility to protect intended victims of a potentially dangerous patient, raises the issue of how to resolve the confidentiality and privilege given to the patient and the protection of the community. A therapist, based on new case law and legislation, may have to change the original treatment plan and include provisions for civil commitment for dangerous patients. A model recommended by Appelbaum in 1985 is based on the Tarasoff case, but is part of any good clinical care and is as follows: First, *assess* potential harm anticipated over the next few days or weeks at most; document in the patient's record. Second, *formulate* a course of action or plan to protect the intended victim (as identified by the patient). This may involve a change or increase of medication, hospitalization, increased security, or warning the intended victim or police; document the course of action. Third, *implement* the plan to protect the victim and document. (*CTP 2119–20. APA 1054, 1081. Har 823–24.*)

77. **(E)** Depression is a side effect of many drugs including antihypertensives (reserpine, beta blockers—propranolol, clonidine), digitalis, alpha-methyl-dopa, steroids (ACTH), hormones (oral contraceptives), antibacterials, analgesics (opiates, ibuprofen, phenacetin), disulfiram, amantadine, levodopa, phenothiazines, phenytoin. Any drug that can deplete catecholamine in the brain may cause depression. (*CTP 631. Har 130.*)

78. (E) It may be hazardous to add a tricyclic to an MAOI treatment; hyperpyrexia and death can occur when both are taken together in high doses. The most common side effect of MAOI is postural hypotension, but MAOI drugs do not affect cardiac conduction. Other common problems are sexual dysfunctions (frequently anorgasmia and impotence), insomnia, and weight gain. When MAOI antidepressants are given with meperidine, seizures, hyperpyrexia, and death can occur (*CTP 1651–52. APA 792, 799. Har 519–20.*)

79. (A) There are three parental preparations of benzodiazepines: chlordiazepoxide, diazepam, and lorazepam. Lorazepam is considered the drug of choice for IV use in seizures and IM use in general. Amitriptyline HCl (10 mg/ml) is available but not usually administered by injection. Fluphenazine decanoate (25 mg/ml) and haloperidol decanoate (50 and 100 mg/ml) are excellent long-acting IM preparations. (*CTP 1580–83. APA 818–19. Har 508, 526–27.*)

80. (B) Nightmares (dream anxiety disorder) and night or sleep terrors (pavor nocturnus, incubus) are parasomnias but are different phenomena. They are seen most often in boys and most start in childhood. A nightmare is a frightening dream that occurs in REM period of sleep (like most other dreams), most often in the second half of the night, and the dream is remembered. Night terror is not a dream, is not remembered but is a frightening arousal state, usually occurring early in the night from stage 3/4 sleep, and is accompanied by autonomic activation, sometimes with movement and sleepwalking. (*CTP 1121–22. Har 166.*)

81. (C) Withdrawal from opioids can be mild with influenza-like reaction such as anxiety, dysphoria, yawning, sweating, fever, rhinorrhea, lacrimation, pupillary dilation, piloerection, hypertension, tachycardia, disrupted sleep, to severe withdrawal symptoms with deep muscle, joint, and abdominal pains, weight loss, and waves of muscle twitching (gooseflesh). (*CTP 649–51. APA 331.*)

82. (E) *AIDS* (acquired immune deficiency syndrome) *dementia* is caused by the HIV III (human immunodeficiency virus) direct involvement of the CNS, causing motor symptoms and intellectual deterioration. The subject may develop associated intracranial tumors (lymphomas), infections (toxoplasmosis), and effects of systemic disease (electrolyte imbalances, septicemia), which can cause mental problems. (*CTP 1306–10. Har 371. APA 290.*)

83. (B) David Malan was influenced by the Tavistock Clinic form of brief psychotherapy. In this psychotherapy, a focal problem to be dealt with in a brief period of time is defined, and a termination date is decided at the start. The more the conflict area manifests itself in the transference, the more positive the outcome; transference interpretations are an important part of the therapeutic process. (*CTP 1564–67. APA 861. Har 591–92.*)

84. (B) *Type I bipolar disorder* is present when one or more manic episodes occur with a history of depressive episodes. The risk of developing a bipolar disorder increases when family members have the disorder (about 60–65% of relatives have a positive history). It starts at an early age (late adolescence or early adulthood, mean age 30), equally divided between males and females, but there is another group, mostly females, whose first episode is in the fifth decade of life. *Bipolar II* (recurrent major depressive episodes, with hypomanic episodes) is two times more frequent in females than in males, and starts at any age, but in 50% of patients the onset is between 20–50 years of age, with a mean of 40 years old. (*CTP 893. APA 414. Har 322.*)

85. (C) Trazodone is the only antidepressant that has the unusual adverse reaction of priapism. Priapism may be irreversible and painful, requiring surgery if erection lasts more than one hour. (*CTP 1647. APA 800. Har 508.*)

86. (A) *Alcohol withdrawal syndrome* should be treated aggressively in the hospital as it can result in convulsions and delirium. Intramuscular thiamine (100 mg) should be given as early as possible especially if Wernicke's syndrome is suspected. Benzodiazepines, especially the long-acting preparations, are safe and effective. Routine administration of phenytoin is not necessary unless there is a history of seizures. If delirium tremens occurs, then phenothiazines or related compounds may be necessary. Usually intravenous fluid replacement is not needed as overhydration may occur. (*CTP 697. Har 709–10. APA 324.*)

87. (E) Anorexia nervosa, bulimia nervosa, and obesity are eating disorders. Anorexia patients have intense fear of gaining weight, are preoccupied with food and being fat, and deny their obvious symptoms. They produce weight loss by reducing total food intake, especially high carbohydrate and fat, and by vigorous exercises, purging activities (self-induced vomiting, laxatives), and diuretic abuse. Amenorrhea can appear before noticeable weight loss. Patients with anorexia nervosa are more likely to have poor sexual adjustment. (*CTP 1854–64. APA 755–56. Har 435.*)

88. (D) Anorexia and bulimia can result in life-threatening medical complications usually following the starvation and the cycling of bingeing and purging. Anorexia nervosa patients develop cardiovascular problems (bradycardia, hypotension, arrhythmias), hematological (anemia, leukopenia), gastrointestinal (delayed gastric

motility, pain, constipation), skeletal changes (osteoporosis), endocrine (hypothyroid-like state, growth failure, amenorrhea), increased blood urea, and peripheral edema. As weight loss becomes more severe, starvation metabolic changes occur with edema, hypotension, bradycardia, and lanugo (appearance of neonatal-like hair). (*CTP 1854–64. Har 436.*)

89. **(C)** *Narcolepsy*, "sleep seizure," is the second most common cause of hypersomnia, occurs equally with men and women, most by age 30, and shows marked familial incidence. There are four distinct features: (1) irresistible impulse for daytime naps, which can occur during work, eating, or driving; (2) cataplexy, a sudden loss of muscle tone; (3) sleep paralysis, occurring just before falling asleep or just after awakening; and (4) hypnagogic hallucinations. Cataplexy should not be confused with catalepsy, which is a trance-like state and a generalized unresponsiveness. Treatment of cataplexy is with stimulants (amphetamine, methylphenidate), and low doses of antidepressant (imipramine, protriptyline), or MAOIs (tranylcypromine). (*CTP 1116–17. Har 123–24. APA 747–48.*)

90. **(B)** *Rapid cycling* is defined as the presence of at least three or four episodes per year. The addition of carbamazepine is often effective in treating this problem, as it potentiates the therapeutic effects of lithium and phenothiazines. An MAO-A inhibitor, clorgyline, not available in the U.S., may be helpful with rapid cyclers. (*CTP 1659–60. APA 431.*)

91. **(A)** Dermatological effects seem to be dose-dependent and include acneform eruptions, follicular and maculopapular eruptions, pretibial ulcerations, worsening of psoriasis, and alopecia. Tetracycline (if used to treat acne, etc.) may cause an increase in retention of lithium and thereby increase toxicity. (Other side effects of lithium therapy are noted in question 73.) (*CTP 1661. APA 821–26. Har 504–5.*)

92. **(A)** The physician should attempt to project passively a sense of being in control. The physician may want to offer medications, food, inquire about patient's concerns, especially about temper, and loss of control. The clinician should not tower over the patient, make sudden moves, stare at or try to force eye contact, and should allow space around the patient. (*CTP 1428–33. APA 1040–41.*)

93. **(D)** The adverse effects of cocaine are similar to those caused by amphetamines. After a binge cycle or chronic use of cocaine, abrupt withdrawal has three symptom phases:

First, during the "crash," which can last up to three or four days, the abuser becomes exhausted from lack of sleep and food, depressed, anxious, insomnic, irritable, with intense craving that decreases.

Second, there are several more days of continued irritability, anxiety, decreased capacity to experience pleasure, excessive sleep, overeating, and continued absence of cocaine craving.

Third, the individual seems to be normalized with normal sleep, better mood, but craving for cocaine becomes intense usually leading to another binge cycle. (*CTP 671–72. Har 421. APA 339–40.*)

94. **(A)** In *functional enuresis*, bedwetting is more common than daytime incontinence. Nocturnal enuresis commonly occurs 30 minutes to three hours after sleep onset. Enuresis is more common in males. Eighty percent of enuretic children have not achieved full bladder control (i.e., primary). Only 1% of enuresis persists into adulthood. About 75% of enuretic children have a first-degree relative with a history of enuresis. Treatment includes appropriate toilet training, especially with the primary form of enuresis, behavioral therapy (classical conditioning with bell and buzzer pad), which is most effective (50%) and safe, pharmacotherapy (i.e., imipramine), which is sometimes effective (30%) but shows a high rate of symptom return during treatment or after cessation of medication, and psychotherapy, which if used alone is not effective. (*CTP 1879–82. APA 690–91.*)

95. **(E)** *Electroconvulsive treatment* (ECT) was first used in the 1930s. It can be the safest (especially with the elderly), least expensive, and a more effective form of treatment. The principal indications for electroconvulsive therapy are severe depression, especially delusional depression, accompanied by changes in vegetative functioning (sleep, appetite, libido) and in activity (psychomotor retardation). Electroconvulsive therapy may also be of benefit for manic excitement not responsive to medications, catatonic schizophrenia, and suicidal behavior. Atypical, neurotic or reactive depressions do not usually respond well to ECT. (*CTP 1676–77. APA 836–37. Har 583–84.*)

96. **(B)** The essential feature of *paranoid personality disorder* is suspiciousness and mistrust of people. The extensive use of projection by these individuals results in their being easily slighted, quick to react with anger, prone to bear grudges, and ready to suspect hidden demeaning or threatening significance in benign remarks or events. These subjects resist treatment. Group therapy is avoided because it involves too much confrontation, behavioral therapies create fear of external control, but nonthreatening, supportive individual psychotherapy may be helpful and tolerated. (*CTP 1365–67. APA 630–31. Har 342.*)

97. **(C)** Most psychiatric disorders are diagnosed more often in males, but elective mutism, somatization disorders, and borderline personality disorder are diagnosed more frequently in females. (*CTP 1833. Har 348.*)

98. **(A)** E. Bleuler defined a fundamental group of symptoms of schizophrenia, the so-called *Bleulerian "Four A's,"* occasionally expanded to five or six. These are *Associations* (thought disorder), *Affect* (blunting), *Autism* (idiosyncratic thinking), and *Ambivalence* (conceptual indecisiveness). The other A's are impaired *Attention* and *Avolition*. Bleuler further stated that delusions and hallucinations were *"Accessory."* (*CTP 586. APA 359. Har 277.*)

99. **(A)** *Phenylketonuria* is an inborn error of metabolism transmitted by an autosomal recessive genetic defect causing a deficiency of phenylalanine hydroxylase. It occurs in 1/10,000–15,000 live births. If untreated by diet early in life (optimally before 3 months of age), severe mental retardation can occur with eczema, vomiting, convulsions (about one-half of cases), erratic and unpredictable behavior, temper tantrums, and autistic-like behaviors. Previously, the urine (which has a musty odor) was tested with ferric chloride: the presence of urinary phenylpyruvic acid in this illness caused a vivid green color. The test had limited sensitivity and false positives. A more reliable test is the Guthrie inhibitor assay, which uses a bacteriological procedure to detect blood phenylalanine. (*CTP 1739, 1741. Har 139.*)

100. **(B)** The *Thematic Apperception Test* (TAT) is an individually administered unstructured or projective test, which assesses personality conflicts, motivation, relationships (individual, family), fantasies, feelings, needs, and conflicts. There are 19–30 cards or scenes of black and white pictures, and one blank card. The shorter version uses 10–12 cards. (*CTP 483–85. APA 1279. Har 54–55.*)